Successfully Surviving a Brain Injury is e ~~~~~~~ and friends. The book nicely covers ~~~~~~~ a positive and helpful perspective. ' ~~~~~~~ done his homework and offers practical inforr of topics, including the emotional aspects of recovery, an important topic which is often neglected.

> *Jeffrey Kreutzer, Ph.D., Professor of Physical Medicine and Rehabilitation, Neurosurgery and Psychiatry, Virginia Commonwealth University*

Every family experiencing brain injury should have *Successfully Surviving a Brain Injury*. It's written in such a personal way. It's so comforting and extremely informative.

> *Tracy Porter, Executive Director of Mothers Against Brain Injury*

Following a traumatic brain injury, family members are in a state of shock and confusion. They are immediately immersed in a medical emergency and emotional crisis that will change their lives forever. This is a much needed book for caregivers as they travel the long complicated and uncertain journey toward recovery with their loved ones.

> *Susan Hansen, COO, San Diego Brain Injury Foundation*

This book is a story of love and devotion and a most helpful guide for the families of a brain injury survivor.

> *Chuck McLafferty, Former President of the Brain Injury Association of South Carolina*

This book is a Godsend to families whose lives have suddenly been affected by a brain injury. The author guides readers through the challenges of recovery, shares valuable information, and provides comfort all at the same time.

> *Deborah D. Palmer, Founder, Brain Injury Connection*

I have worked with hundreds of individuals with traumatic brain injury and family members, and I know that *Successfully Surviving a Brain Injury* represents a reality that so many people face.

> *Deborah Delgado, Traumatic Brain Injury Project Director for the Disability Rights Network of Pennsylvania*

I wish this book had been available when my husband was injured. Having the term "brain injury" thrown at me with nothing to explain it was terrifying. Garry Prowe spoke with many survivors and caregivers. He tells the story of all of us, and he tells it well.

> *Cindy Reed, Tampa, Florida*

The world of brain injury is foreign and scary. I wish we had *Successfully Surviving a Brain Injury* after our son's injury. There are many books on the medical aspects of brain injury, but few about the emotions that accompany it. The assurance that these feelings are normal is so helpful! I hope every critical care hospital has copies of this book.

Deanna Kritch, Elmira, Oregon

My son sustained a brain injury and we were numb as we walked in the fog. *Successfully Surviving a Brain Injury* would have made such a huge difference in our understanding of brain injury. Most important of all, it would have given us some very much needed hope. The doctors and nurses do not have the time to even come close to imparting the information contained in this book.

Judith Hacks, Ontario, Canada

We have undergone the heartache, stress, hope, and discouragement of our son's brain injury for nearly six years. Garry Prowe truly understands brain injury. Not only has he lived it, but he has interviewed many others who shared their stories with him.

Dee Strickland Johnson, Phoenix, Arizona

I would have given anything to have a book like *Successfully Surviving a Brain Injury* when we were stumbling our way through the days, weeks, and months of dealing with my son's traumatic brain injury. It is so complete and easy to understand.

Joan Dunham, St. Petersburg, Florida

Successfully Surviving a Brain Injury gives hope to survivors by providing answers to questions we either can't get out due to our injury or don't even know to ask. The most important thing I learned is that the survivor is never going to be the person he was before his injury. But that doesn't mean he still can't be a contributing member of society.

Dave McGuire, 3-year survivor, Vancouver, Canada

Successfully Surviving a Brain Injury deals so well with the emotional issues of living with a brain injury that other books skim over or ignore completely. Even the darkest clouds have a silver lining. But it takes exceptional people like Garry Prowe to help others look beyond the darkness.

Jode Webster, 18-year survivor, Gisborne, New Zealand

Successfully Surviving A Brain Injury

A Family Guidebook

Brain Injury Success Books

Successfully Surviving a Brain Injury

A Family Guidebook

From the Emergency Room to Selecting a Rehabilitation Facility

Garry Prowe

Foreword by

Susan H. Connors
President & CEO
Brain Injury Association of America

Brain Injury Success Books

Publisher's Cataloging-in-Publication Data

Prowe, Garry
  Successfully surviving a brain injury: a family guidebook, from the emergency room to selecting a rehabilitation facility; Garry Prowe; foreword by Susan H. Connors.
    p. cm.
  Series: Successfully surviving a brain injury : a family guidebook
  Includes bibliographical references and index.
  ISBN 978-0-9841974-3-9
  1. Brain injury--Patients--Rehabilitation. 2. Brain--Wounds and injuries--Patients--Rehabilitation. 3. Brain Injuries--rehabilitation. 4. Brain damage. 5. Brain damage--Patients--Biography. 6. Brain--Wounds and injuries--Patients--Family relationships. I. Connors, Susan H. II. Series. III. Title.
  RD594 .P76 2010
  617.4/81044—dc22   2009934999

First edition 2010
Published by Brain Injury Success Books
www.BrainInjurySuccess.org

Note: The contents of this book are, to the best of our knowledge, true, complete, and current. However, certain statements may be outdated or inaccurate. This book is presented as a general starting point for addressing the myriad issues related to a brain injury. It should not replace or conflict with the advice of medical, legal, financial, insurance, and other professionals. The information is offered with no guarantees on the part of the author or Brain Injury Success Books. The author and publisher disclaim all liability in connection with the use of this book.

This book is available at a special discount to organizations that support survivors of a brain injury and their families. For more information, email Info@BrainInjurySuccess.org or call 352-672-6672.

To my sisters Barbara

Barbara Prowe

&

Barbara First

Thank you.

Table of Contents

Foreword 13

Acknowledgements.. 15

1. Introduction.. 17

2. How to Use This Book 27

3. A Momentary Lapse of Attention 31

4. Brain Injury Basics #1..37

    The Healthy Brain 38
    The Injured Brain 39
    The Healing Brain 45

5. The Litany of Uncertainty.. 47

6. Brain Injury Basics #2 53

    Dealing with Doctors 54
    The Glasgow Coma Scale 57
    What Is a Coma? 59
    The Rancho Los Amigos Scale.. 64

Checklist #1 - The First Few Days...................................68

7. A Tsunami of Emotions.. 71

8. How to Succeed as a Caregiver...........................79

    Take Care of Yourself 80
    Faith 91
    Asking for Help..92
    The Family and Medical Leave Act...................95
    Case Managers...98
    How Well Will My Survivor Recover?...............101

Checklist #2 - Focus on What You Can Control.............. 105

9. Waiting, Watching, Hoping............................. 107

10. Paying the Bills...115

    Health Insurance 115
    Disability Pay.. 123
    Disability Pay & Health Insurance for Children........... 134
    Do We Need an Attorney? 139

Checklist #3 - Paying the Bills 146

11. Trapped in the Fog...................................... 149

12. Life with a Brain Injury 157

    Physical Impairments 159
    Cognitive Impairments 160
    Communication Impairments 163
    Emotional Impairments.................................. 164
    Behavioral Impairments 164
    Social Impairments 166
    Spasticity 167
    Seizures 169
    The Impact of Brain Injury on the Family.....................171

Checklist #4 - Preparing Yourself and Your Family......... 178

13. In Limbo......181

14. An Introduction to Rehabilitation............... 187

    Post-Traumatic Amnesia............... 187
    Rehabilitation Basics...................... 192
    Selecting a Rehabilitation Facility............... 196
    Nursing Homes............206

Checklist #5 - Planning for Rehabilitation...................... 209

15. Eleven Years Later......211

Glossary...................... 219

List of Essential Resources............... 229

State Brain Injury Associations 234

Index 235

11

Foreword

Traumatic brain injury statistics in the United States are staggering: 1.4 million people sustain an injury *each year*; 50,000 people die. The economic cost is a whopping $60 billion annually. These numbers indicate the scope of the issue, but they don't tell the real story. The real stories are both heartwarming and heart-wrenching. Once told, they forever change how we view brain injury and the issues that surround it.

Most people don't understand brain injury. If they are familiar with the term at all, they think of brain injury as an event—often an accident—for which the victim is treated in a hospital and then released home to live his or her life. This is far from the real story.

Many people who sustain brain injuries never go to the hospital; when they eventually seek medical care, the injury is often misdiagnosed. Those who are admitted to the hospital, often with moderate to severe injuries, may be slow to recover or may not recover fully. For some, brain injury is a disease causative or a disease-accelerative, ushering an onslaught of neurologic and neuroendocrine disorders, bowel, bladder and sexual dysfunction, and sometimes psychiatric disease.

Just as every individual is different, every brain injury is different. But every injury affects the entire family. Understanding brain injury is the first step to regaining control over the many challenges brain injury presents. Understanding brain injury is also crucial to becoming an effective caregiver and advocate. This book offers useful insights into the challenges families face along with helpful advice. The Brain Injury Association of America is grateful to people like Garry and Jessica, who have faced this life-changing event and are willing to share their experience with others.

Founded in 1980, the Brain Injury Association of America (BIAA) is the voice of brain injury. We are dedicated to increasing access to quality health care and raising awareness and understanding of brain injury through advocacy, education, and research. With a nationwide network of more than forty chartered state affiliates, as well as hundreds of local chapters and support groups across the country, the Brain Injury Association of America provides help, hope, and healing for individuals who live with brain injury, their families, and the professionals who serve them. To learn more about brain injury, please visit our Web site at www.biausa.org or call our National Brain Injury Information Center at 800-444-6443.

Susan H. Connors, President/CEO
Brain Injury Association of America
September 2009

Acknowledgements

To Joanne Lozar Glenn, thank you for giving me invaluable advice and the confidence to write this book. To Susan H. Connors, Harvey Jacobs, Marilyn Lash, Bob Cluett, Jeffrey Kreutzer, Suzanne Minnich, Dorothy Cronin, June O'Donal, Deborah Delgado, John Kumpf, Howard Barkin, Scott LaPoint, Kenneth Kolpan, and Lawrence Lottenberg for supporting my work just when I needed a boost.

Thank you to the 300 members of my panel of survivors, caregivers, and professionals. Without your participation, this project would not exist.

While I hesitate to name names due to the certainty of my overlooking someone on the panel who worked especially hard to support this project, I'll do it anyway. The folks listed below deserve a special note of gratitude. To those particularly diligent panel members who I have unconscionably omitted, I ask for your forgiveness.

The survivors on the panel who were exceptionally helpful include Anne Forrest, Alison Schiebelhut, John Onorato, Ann Boriskie, Ann Carter, Barbara de Catanzano, Jenny Ayers, Bernie Goggins, Bettina Rose Hughes, Deborah Palmer, Bruce Traub, Sandy Archer, Celeste Palmer, Candy Gustafson, Dave McGuire, Christy Marcondes, Melissa Baker, David Moore, Diane Quimby, Tracy Tarvers, Paul Harpin, Iadora Kelley, Jack Sisson, Jason Ferguson, Joseph Dilullo, Jamie Crawford, Jode Webster, Jessica Baldwin, Jennifer Hannah, Jim Eastman, Julia Pratt, Jan Zbynski, Kathy Hay, Kim Winter, Elizabeth Merkley, Louise Matthewson, Thomas Kelley, Marilou Fallis, Les Paul Morgan, Dick Ohmart, Laurie Deptula, Nadia Nadiak, Georgia Pritchard, Pam Hayes, Alicia Payne, Jennifer Pilon, Rebekah Vandergriff, David Dermer, Richard De Pol, Shane Becker,

Ryan Holland, Sarah Rose Stewart, Janet Blair, Vicki Cote, and Vycki Fleming.

The caregivers who contributed the most include Carole Thorpe, Bonnie Slager, Christine Ritchie, Tracy Porter, Denise Bryant, Dodie Sullivan, Frances Bloch, Gail Groninger, Helen Cloud, Jan Verrinder, Kathie Sell, Donna Lewis, Cindy Reed, Chuck McClafferty, Monika Ellis, Pat Moss, Martha Burnham, Susan Hansen, Sharon Huey, Tracey Clothier, Chris Wales, Dee Strickland Johnson, Olga Sowchuk, Connie Koebke, Deanna Kritch, Debra Gordon, Dorothy Mathers, Judith Hacks, Sue Stauffer, Joan Dunham, Kathie Stroehlein, Tanya Ison, Anne Zusselman, and Marguerite McKinney.

While these panel members have been a tremendous help, answering my many questions and reviewing early drafts of this book, I alone am responsible for any errors.

Many thanks to family and friends who reviewed and commented upon the manuscript, especially Barbara Prowe, Don Helin, Elliot Yasmer, and Kathy First.

Thank you, Jennifer Prowe for the cover artwork and your enthusiastic support from beginning to end.

My gratitude to my copy editor Starlyn First, who rescued me from some embarrassing punctuation, grammar, and typos.

Finally, thank you Jessica, for showing me every day how to live successfully with adversity.

1

Introduction

You are reading this book because someone you love has suffered a brain injury. The form, extent, and consequences of the damage are yet unknown. Her doctors are unable to make a prognosis. "Every brain injury is unique and unpredictable," they say. "It will be months before we know for sure." A hospital social worker has advised you to hope for the best, but prepare for the worst.

This news is incomprehensible. What does the social worker mean by "the worst"? What must you do to "be prepared"? When will your spouse emerge from her coma? How badly will she be impaired by her brain injury? How soon will her doctors speak with some certainty? How will this misfortune impact your family and your future?

In 1997, I was in your place. My wife, Jessica, suffered a serious brain injury in an automobile accident. Like you, I was relieved to hear that she would survive her near-death experience. Like you, I was devastated to learn that she would acquire any number of lifelong impairments. And, like you, I had many questions and few answers. "Only time will tell," her doctors repeated over and over. Confusion, panic, grief, and fatigue were my constant companions every hour of every day for weeks.

I longed for some cause to be hopeful. I had to believe that survivors of traumas like Jessica's recover well. I craved examples of people with serious brain injuries living full and happy lives.

You should be comforted to know that people do recover successfully from a brain injury, and neither a miracle nor a superhuman effort is required. Jessica and countless others are living proof of this. Despite her considerable disabilities, my wife has created a new life that is full of love and joy, challenges and rewards, family and friends.

To Succeed, You Must Change Your Mind

First and foremost, you must understand that a successful recovery from a serious brain injury is not a full recovery. All but a handful of charmed survivors spend the rest of their lives challenged—mildly, moderately, or severely—by their brain injury.

These challenges—by themselves—do not make for an unsuccessful recovery. Success is cut short when the inevitable impairments caused by a serious brain injury are denied or not accommodated by both the survivor *and* those around her.

The single most important element to achieving a successful recovery is a clear understanding of your goal. Jessica's car crash caused irreparable damage to her brain. She was transformed in many ways. To succeed in her recovery, Jessica needed to "change her mind." She needed to acknowledge and learn to live with her new deficits. She needed to alter the way she viewed herself. She needed to adjust her life goals.

A successful recovery also demands that the people surrounding the survivor be understanding, compassionate, and accommodating. They must change the way they view her. They must learn how their survivor has been impaired, and how they can work with her to compensate for these new deficits.

They must strive to understand—without frustration, anger, or resentment—that the unwelcome transformations in their survivor are symptoms of her brain injury, not conscious choices or failures of character.

This is far from easy. The other day, for example, more than eleven years after Jessica's accident, I doubted her efforts as we paid the monthly bills. I was eager to complete that chore and return to writing this book. When Jessica asked for basic instruction in revising spreadsheets on our computer—for the one-thousandth time—my frustration overwhelmed my reason. I unjustly and robustly accused her of laziness. But Jessica wasn't negligent. She couldn't recall how to work with spreadsheets because her brain injury has compromised both her memory and her ability to grasp new information.

Jessica's recovery is successful—in no small part—because we accepted the unwelcome reality that she was transformed forever by her brain injury. Without this acknowledgement, Jessica and I would have had unreasonable goals. Expecting a person with a serious brain injury to return to her previous self is a sure-fire path to failure.

To achieve a successful recovery, you must "change your mind."

Mild, Moderate, and Severe Brain Injuries

There are three levels of brain injury: mild, moderate, and severe. Mild injuries are by far the most common. They cover a broad range of outcomes. The majority are, indeed, mild. They usually are shaken off and rarely given a second thought. Some mild injuries, however, are cruelly mislabeled. A mild brain injury can leave someone so infirmed, she is unable to return to work or school, or live independently. Multiple mild injuries— such as the concussions endured by boxers and football players—can result in considerable cumulative brain damage.

At the other extreme is a subset of severe brain injuries called catastrophic. Survivors of catastrophic trauma are either in a vegetative state or so impaired they are unable to set goals for themselves to achieve a better recovery or to improve the quality of their lives.

In this book, I address the injuries that fall between these two extremes: the mildest of the mild and the catastrophic. For the sake of simplicity, I call them "serious brain injuries."

Warning: These labels are easily misinterpreted. If one is said to have a mild brain injury, people may expect a complete recovery. If she is diagnosed with a severe injury, people may expect little improvement. Both assumptions are premature, often inaccurate, and potentially harmful to the survivor's recovery. Jessica's brain injury is severe. Yet, she has made considerable progress in her rehabilitation and recovery. She now enjoys a full life and enhances the lives of those around her.

Every Brain Injury Is Unique ...

Every brain injury varies in the type, location, and extent of the damage suffered. Consequently, each survivor acquires a unique mix of symptoms. One person, for example, may need a cane to compensate for her shaky balance and the patience of others to comprehend her slurred speech. A second survivor may display no physical complaints, but explodes with anger when asked to take out the garbage. She also strikes up long, one-sided conversations with strangers. A third person may be unable to find the right word in conversation and becomes agitated in public places. She just wants to be left alone to play video games in her room. A fourth survivor may display no outward signs of an injury, but has subtle lapses of concentration and information processing, which only those closest to her can recognize.

.... But the Stages of Recovery Are the Same

While each survivor is affected uniquely by her brain injury, all strive toward the same milestones of recovery. They are the ten levels of the *Rancho Los Amigos Scale of Cognitive Functioning*. The Rancho Scale is commonly used to describe the condition of a brain injury patient. It begins at Level 1, when the survivor is in a deep coma. It ends at Level 10, when she is acting independently, purposefully, and appropriately. Please don't be intimidated by the awkward title of this handy tool. Soon, you will be as familiar with the ten levels of the Rancho Scale as you are with the symptoms of the common cold.

It is important to recognize that the road to recovery often has detours and dead ends. Some survivors progress quickly. Others advance a level or two, then regress before advancing again. Many fail to move beyond a certain level. How your survivor works her way through the Rancho levels cannot be predicted. This uncertainty is one of the agonies of brain injury.

Jessica traveled through the Rancho levels in textbook fashion. Consequently, our story may provide a roadmap of the journey you are about to take through the bewildering world of brain injury.

Benefiting from the Experiences of Many

As I tell our story, I examine my actions over the past eleven years from a more informed perspective. Throughout Jessica's recovery and rehabilitation, I often felt as though I were barely hanging in there, certainly not succeeding. As I look back, I frequently wonder, "Why didn't I think of that?" or "Why didn't somebody tell me that?"

My experiences—while instructive—are the experiences of just one caregiver. To better understand how survivors and their family members overcome the challenges of recovering from a brain injury and creating a fulfilling new life, I assembled a panel of brain injury veterans. The members of this panel include more than 150 people living with a brain injury, 110 family caregivers, and forty medical professionals. I posed countless questions to these brain injury experts and benefited enormously from their generous participation.

Absorbing and acting upon the information and advice I have compiled in this book will make your efforts to support your survivor more effective.

I also hope that this book will inspire you to persevere when you are overwhelmed and disheartened by the many obstacles you will encounter on the road to a successful recovery.

Helping your survivor recover successfully may be the most rewarding job of your life.

Seven Reasons to Be Encouraged

First, brain injuries are far more common than you may imagine. Medical professionals often call brain injury a "silent epidemic." According to the Centers for Disease Control and Prevention, 1.4 million Americans sustain a traumatic brain injury each year. *The Journal of Head Trauma Rehabilitation* reports that an estimated 3.17 million Americans live with a long-term disability related to a traumatic brain injury.

These figures do not include the many other causes of brain injury, such as heart attack, stroke, aneurysm, tumor, infection, substance abuse, near-drowning, and electrical shock. Each year, far more cases of brain injury occur than those of breast cancer, multiple sclerosis, spinal cord injury, and HIV/AIDS combined.

Second, the wars in Iraq and Afghanistan have placed brain injury on the front page of newspapers and magazines. As many as one in six combatants in these conflicts suffer brain trauma. These often gravely wounded warriors provide the medical world added motivation to develop more effective protocols and rehabilitative therapies to treat brain injury.

Third, recent research has discovered that the injured brain has the adaptability to reorganize itself to compensate for the damaged areas. This remarkable ability is known as *plasticity*. In practical terms, plasticity enables survivors to recover—via intensive therapy—some of the abilities lost to their injury.

Fourth, developments in stem cell research also are heartening. Theoretically, stem cells can be transplanted into an injured portion of the brain and then regenerate into the type of cells that have been destroyed. While the harvesting of stem cells from embryos is controversial, new stem cell sources— bone marrow, blood from placentas, skin, and non-viable embryos—are being studied.

Fifth, innovations in a relatively new field of therapy— *cognitive rehabilitation*—are producing promising results in restoring not only a survivor's ability to concentrate, remember, and solve problems, but also her capacity to reenter the community and to enjoy a more satisfying life.

Sixth, new technologies, such as voice recognition computer software and sophisticated electronic devices, designed to help busy people everywhere perform their daily activities faster and better, also are helping the disabled live more independent lives.

Finally, there are many organizations ready to guide you and your survivor toward a more successful recovery. From the Brain Injury Association of America (800-444-6443 & www.biausa.org) and its state affiliates to federal, state, and local government agencies; community support groups; and peer mentors; experienced and knowledgeable people are waiting for your call.

Warnings, Apologies, and Notes

First, I have spent many hours in hospitals and other medical facilities observing and interacting with doctors, nurses, and therapists, but I'm not a medical professional. My intent is not to offer you medical advice; it is to make you a more educated consumer of medical, government, financial, insurance, case management, and legal services.

Second, the science of medicine and the protocols for treating brain injury are advancing rapidly. Major reforms in health care are being considered in the United States. Insurance, legal, and government policies and procedures change often. While I have strived to be 100 percent accurate with the information I present in this book, some statements are likely to become outdated quickly.

Third, recovering from a brain injury is a harrowing experience for both the survivor and the caregiver. Unless you have taken copious notes, your memory can be clouded by time and tainted by the grief, confusion, fear, and fatigue you felt at the time. Consequently, my depictions of the characters in this story—doctors, nurses, therapists, administrators, social workers, family, friends, and colleagues—may be unduly harsh. For this, I apologize. To avoid embarrassing anyone, including myself, I use fictitious names for all medical and administrative personnel.

Fourth, a welcome development in terminology for people living with a disability is person-first language. Rather than saying "a brain-injured person," it is preferable to say "a person living with a brain injury." Folks living with a brain injury are people first, with the countless characteristics that make each of us unique. Just one of these characteristics—albeit a major one—is their brain injury.

A large majority of the panel members living with a brain injury, however, dislike person-first language. They prefer to be called survivors. They wear this label as a badge of the courage and determination they display every day of their lives.

Therefore, to indicate a person living with a brain injury, I primarily use the term "survivor." For variety, I also use the terms "individual," "person," "loved one," and "patient." For brevity, I generally avoid the much longer term "person living with a brain injury." I apologize to those offended by this choice.

Fifth, a word regarding my use of gender pronouns: I find the construct "she/he" awkward, and alternating between "she" and "he" is confusing. Since in our story Jessica is the survivor and I am the caregiver, I portray the person living with a brain injury as female and the caregiver as male throughout the book. Please do not view this choice as gender stereotyping. A large majority of people living with a brain injury are male.

Sixth, if you would like to learn more about the *Successfully Surviving a Brain Injury* project, please visit our Web site at www.BrainInjurySuccess.org. Here you can read reviews of our favorite brain-injury books and some of our articles.

Finally, if you find any inaccuracies in this book, if you would like to comment on its contents, if you would like to participate in this project as a panel member, or if you would like to suggest topics to be covered in future volumes of this series, please email me at Info@BrainInjurySuccess.org. I look forward to hearing from you.

Notes

2

How to Use This Book

This book has a number of distinct parts. If you are a brain injury novice, like I was, I suggest you read or at least skim through the entire text. I have packed a lot of information onto these pages. You may be surprised to discover a topic that at first glance seems unrelated to your situation but, upon further consideration, turns out to be quite helpful. For example, you may dismiss the idea of hiring a case manager or an attorney until you see how these professionals can make your life easier at a difficult time.

The *odd-numbered chapters* of the book recount the first twenty-three days of Jessica's recovery. This includes:

- Her medical treatment in the emergency room and the intensive care unit
- Our long days at the hospital waiting apprehensively for Jessica to emerge from her coma
- Our shock and distress over her infant-like and bizarre behavior as she awoke from her coma
- The early stages of my education in becoming a more effective caregiver and advocate for Jessica

For certain readers, only portions of the story—such as Jessica's gradual awakening or her struggles to make sense of her new world—will be of interest. Other readers will want to follow Jessica's story closely, using it as a rough guide to their survivor's recovery.

Throughout Jessica's recovery, I often felt that I was trapped in a maze of time-gobbling, energy-sapping, urgent, and complicated insurance, financial, medical, legal, family, and personal matters, such as health insurance, disability income, and selecting a rehabilitation facility for Jessica. I had too many questions and too few answers to perform these crucial tasks well. I spent far too much time surfing the Internet, making phone calls, and wandering through libraries and bookstores searching for the information I lacked.

I constantly worried that I might overlook something critical or make a mistake that would deny Jessica the benefits due her and, possibly, undermine our financial future.

The *even-numbered chapters* of this book are a series of stand-alone essays presenting the practical information and advice I collected to help you complete these chores quickly and accurately. These brief, easy-to-read essays will:

- Educate you in the basics of brain injury and explain why—with only a handful of exceptions—recovery from a serious brain injury always is incomplete
- Give you an overview of the early stages of the recovery process
- Suggest ways to make this stressful and exhausting time easier for you and your family
- Tell you what you need to know about health insurance and disability pay
- Describe how a case manager and an attorney can assist you
- Prepare you for the next stage of your patient's recovery: rehabilitation

- Summarize the wide range of potential impairments your survivor may suffer as a consequence of her brain injury
- Give you a glimpse of the future by identifying the factors that influence how well someone recovers from a serious brain injury

The third part of this book—the *Checklists for Success*—is a series of five handy checklists designed to help you identify and manage those thorny and time-consuming insurance, financial, medical, legal, family, and personal matters. The checklists are located on pages 68, 105, 146, 178, and 209.

I have tried to make this book easy to read, using words familiar to most everyone. At times, though, I introduce medical terms. You will hear this language regularly and should become comfortable with it. When you come across an unfamiliar word, go to the *Glossary*, where I define and explain how these terms relate to a brain injury. Please, don't be put off by this medical lingo; with a little effort, it will soon become part of your everyday vocabulary.

I also have tried to anticipate and answer the questions you have now, as well as those you will have in the weeks and months ahead. I'm certain, however, that I have not answered all of your questions completely. In the *List of Essential Resources*, I recommend a small group of organizations and books that you can—in this age of information overload—trust to provide accurate and accessible information.

Notes

3

A Momentary Lapse of Attention
A Brain Is Injured

It was an unseasonably cool early September morning. Jessica and I woke to a clamoring alarm clock, accompanied by the persistent meowing of five hungry kitties. In my thin pajamas, I shivered when I opened the door to collect the *Washington Post* from the front stoop.

Jessica showered and dressed quickly, skipped breakfast, hurriedly kissed me goodbye, and rushed out the door. She expected yet another hectic day at the office. She was eager to be at her desk before the first crisis developed.

Jessica and her colleagues maintained the administrative computing system at a small university. The academic year had begun the previous week. The new computer software, installed and thoroughly tested throughout the summer, revealed its inevitable flaws in real-life conditions. Student registration and billing, dormitory room assignments, parking and meal passes, and last-minute revisions to university procedures pushed the new software and its overseers to the max. Unexpected problems—if not handled at once—threatened to bring chaos to the campus.

I knew Jessica's first stop would be the local diner for her morning jolt of caffeine, an iced tea with lots of lemon. To get there, she had to cross a divided highway, clogged with politicians, civil servants, diplomats, lobbyists, and military personnel scurrying into our nation's capital.

The survivors of serious brain injuries are unable to recall the events that transform their lives. The shock to their brain temporarily prevents any memories from being stored. So, we can only guess what Jessica was thinking when she made her nearly fatal mistake. She probably was mulling over the work awaiting her: the papers piled on her desk, the constantly ringing telephone, the administrative fires in need of dousing.

As Jessica waited to cross the highway, a white minivan pulled up on her left, blocking her view of the two southbound lanes. A moment later, the minivan inched forward for a closer look at the oncoming traffic. Jessica might have interpreted this move as a sign that the road was clear. Whatever the reason, she drove into the path of a rapidly approaching behemoth, a Ford Expedition.

This single, momentary lapse of attention changed our lives forever.

The SUV driver, shocked by the sudden appearance of a vehicle in his path, had little time to react. He zigged left when zagging right would have been a better choice. He smashed into the driver's side of our much smaller Honda Accord, propelling it across the low concrete median into one of the two northbound lanes which, thanks to a timely red light, were vacant.

The powerful force of the collision between the two mismatched vehicles triggered the rapid acceleration and deceleration of Jessica's brain. Floating in a pool of cerebro-spinal fluid, it bounced from side to side within her more stationary skull, like a ping-pong ball in a lottery drawing. The portions of her brain that slammed against the rough edges of the inside of her skull were badly bruised. They began to swell and bleed.

As Jessica lay unconscious, pinned inside the crumpled car, crucial minutes were ticking away. Trauma specialists speak of the *golden hour*, referring to the sixty minutes that elapse after a major injury. Receiving expert medical treatment within this golden hour often means the difference between life and death. This is particularly true for victims of a brain injury. As time passes, the damage to their brain can escalate, often fatally, until preventive measures are taken.

Emergency vehicles reached the scene ten minutes after the accident, an amazing feat in the congested commuter traffic of our Washington, D.C. suburb. When the rescue squad arrived, they found a totaled sedan, a critically injured driver, and traffic backed up for miles.

Once the rescue squad freed Jessica from the wreck, they assessed her neurological condition. They employed the *Glasgow Coma Scale* (GCS), a universal, quick, and easy-to-calculate measure of the gravity of a brain injury. Jessica's GCS score of four indicated a severe trauma.

When the ambulance screeched to a halt at the emergency room doors, the trauma team, assembled and waiting, went to work. Their priority was to prevent, or at least minimize, any secondary damage to Jessica's brain.

Think for a moment about the contents of your skull. The brain consumes about eighty percent of the space. The rest is filled with three thin protective membranes and cerebrospinal fluid, which cleanses and cushions the brain.

Inside Jessica's skull, traumatized brain tissue was swelling and bleeding, crowding the space usually occupied by fluid. This was creating stress within her skull, known by doctors as *intracranial pressure* or *ICP*. As the ICP in this confined area increased, healthy brain tissue was being pushed into and torn and bruised by the bony ridges of the interior surface of her skull. This was causing additional swelling, bleeding, and even more pressure. This perilous cascade of secondary damage was threatening Jessica's life.

When the rigid skull allows no more room for blood and swollen tissue, the only outlet is the brainstem, which attaches the brain to the spinal cord. If too much weight pushed down on Jessica's brainstem—the regulator of vital processes, such as breathing, digestion, and heartbeat—she would die.

To measure Jessica's ICP, the trauma team implanted a device—called an intracranial pressure monitor—into her skull, just below her hairline. Detecting excess pressure within the skull and acting quickly to relieve it saves many lives.

As the trauma team raced to preserve Jessica's life and minimize further havoc to her brain, I was blissfully ignorant of the events unfolding.

I had placed the day's newspaper atop the recycling pile and dove into a mound of my medical bills. I was home, as usual, on this workday, having retired eighteen months earlier due to disabling chronic pain.

The telephone rang. The caller identified himself as Tom, a social worker assigned to the intensive care unit (ICU) at a nearby hospital. His words, "car accident," "serious condition," and "get here as soon as possible" staggered me. I demanded more information.

"What are her injuries? How badly is she hurt? Is she dying?"

Tom professionally deflected my frantic questions.

"I'm not a doctor. I don't know the details of her condition," he said. "You should get here right away."

I hung up the phone and raced around the house, trying to identify what I would need at the hospital. The one essential item—our address book filled with phone numbers—escaped my attention. I felt a knot of panic expanding in my chest. This painful tangle of anxiety and fear would be my companion, unraveling bit by bit over the next few months as I learned to cope with Jessica's injury.

When I regained my composure, I called a cab and then waited, striding back and forth across the living room, my eyes all the time on the windswept, empty street outside. The oldest and wisest of our cats seemed to know something awful had happened. She attempted to comfort me, but in my distress, I brushed her aside. I tried to remain calm, aware that I might soon be called on to make crucial decisions about Jessica's medical care. Despite my pleas to the dispatcher that I had an emergency, thirty excruciating minutes passed before the taxi arrived. I was bursting with fear and impatience and my lower back was throbbing from my nervous pacing.

The cab drove me past the scene of Jessica's collision. I saw our car, reconfigured into a pile of scrap metal. *How could anyone survive such a wreck?* I thought. My first question to the social worker, who met me at the emergency room (ER) door, was "Is she alive?"

Tom led me to the ICU, a bright, surprisingly quiet area, the size of a basketball court. The nurses' station on the left was bustling with doctors annotating charts and nurses dashing to and fro. A harried clerk was handling phone calls from anguished family members—soon to include more than a few of ours—anxious for updates on their loved one's condition. The twelve patient rooms, each enclosed with a glass door, windows, and blinds, occupied the entire right side of the unit.

In the first cubicle, Jessica rested peacefully. Her eyes were closed. Except for the slight up-and-down movement of her chest, she was motionless. What grabbed my attention and wouldn't let go was the intracranial pressure monitor drilled into her forehead. I would spend much of the next week nervously watching the screen displaying Jessica's ICP.

I took her limp hand into my jittery one and scanned the jumble of medical paraphernalia keeping Jessica alive. A ventilator was pumping oxygen into her lungs through a tube in her mouth, freeing her body of the taxing act of breathing. A second tube, threaded through Jessica's nose, emptied her stomach to prevent vomiting. Later, this tube would be used to feed her. A cervical collar held her neck stiff. Her left leg was in traction. Needles and plastic tubing, wires and electrodes covered much of her body. Bags of medications and fluids dangled from metal stands. A pouch collecting urine hung on the side of her bed. She wore elastic stockings to guard against blood clots.

An assortment of machines, flashing numbers and displaying wave patterns, clicked and beeped, filling the silence between us. (For days, I was fearful that one of these contraptions—especially the ICP monitor—would blare that something was terribly wrong.)

A nurse permitted me to sit with Jessica for just ten minutes. When I reluctantly left, Tom guided me to a small, comfortably furnished room just outside the ICU. This closet-of-a-space provides the families of new patients the privacy to adjust to the precarious condition of their loved one. In other words, it's a place where you can cry without embarrassment.

When Tom left me alone, I took advantage of the privacy. The images of the twisted wreckage of our car, Jessica lying motionless in bed, and the ICP monitor bored into her forehead fed my misery.

But I was grateful for two things. Jessica was alive and, remarkably, she had been wheeled into the emergency room with five minutes of her golden hour to spare.

4

Brain Injury Basics #1
A Brain Injury Is Forever

For those without medical training, trying to comprehend the intricate operations of the brain can seem overwhelming. Rest assured; it's not necessary for a devoted caregiver to know how the brain works and what happens when it is injured, especially during the tense, confusing, and exhausting first few days or weeks after an injury. If you would rather not puzzle your way through the operations of the brain, feel free to skip this chapter. Doing so will not diminish your understanding of the rest of the book.

For readers seeking a basic knowledge of the brain, this chapter describes:

- How the healthy brain works
- What happens when the brain is injured
- How the brain heals
- Why this healing is incomplete
- How survivors contribute to the healing of their injured brains

The Healthy Brain

The human brain is three pounds of a grooved, pinkish-gray, walnut-shaped, jelly-like substance. As vulnerable to sticks and stones as Jell-O, our most vital organ is guarded by four layers of defense.

The brain floats in a nourishing and cleansing pool of liquid called *cerebrospinal fluid*. Wrapped around the brain and bathed by this fluid are three sheet-like, shock-absorbing membranes or *meninges*, which extend down through the body with the spinal cord. Enclosing the brain and the meninges are the eight, quarter-inch-thick skull bones. These bones are covered by muscles, skin, hair, the occasional hat, and—not nearly often enough—a helmet.

The brain houses a complex network of billions of microscopic nerve cells called *neurons*. Each neuron, which is separated from its neighbors by an infinitesimal gap, has three parts. We need only be familiar with the long, wiry *axon*, which transmits signals to and from adjacent neurons.

When you wake up with a yawn, ponder the day ahead, smell the coffee brewing, stretch your muscles, and climb out of bed, signals speed from one neuron to the next, propelled by an electrical pulse that triggers the release of chemicals known as *neurotransmitters*. The possible pathways for nerve messages circulating at unfathomable speed around the brain are endless, some sixty trillion. They rearrange themselves constantly as we go about our daily activities.

⤏ Located at the base of the brain is a mass of thick nerve fibers called the *brainstem*. It connects the brain to the spinal cord, which passes messages between the body and the brain. The brainstem also houses the control centers of those activities that usually occur automatically, such as breathing, heartbeat, digestion, and, of particular note for our purposes, arousal or consciousness.

The brain is nourished by blood—which contains oxygen—through four arteries at its base. If one artery becomes blocked or damaged, the other three expand to maintain a sufficient flow of blood and oxygen. The brain is harmed by a lack of blood and oxygen much faster than any other body part. Without oxygen, neurons die.

Each component of the brain has its unique role. Matching the areas of the brain to their particular functions demands a degree of medical terminology and explanation beyond this elementary discussion.

Our more complex abilities, such as speech and memory, are performed by two or more components cooperating. For example, the brain has no single memory center. Our memories likely are stored as pathways among the billions of neurons.

After hours of reading about brain injury, I can't match Jessica's deficits with the damaged portions of her brain. This is not to say that physicians are unable to predict likely impairments based on the location and gravity of an injury. What I'm suggesting is that caregivers without a medical degree be cautious in making their own prognoses.

The Injured Brain

Most brain injuries are caused by some form of trauma, such as a car collision, a bicycle accident, a gunshot wound, an assault, a sports mishap, a fall, or the concussive blast of an improvised explosive device on the battlefields of Iraq and Afghanistan. These are called *traumatic brain injuries* or *TBIs*.

There are two types of traumatic brain injury: (1) *closed head* and (2) *open head*. Sometimes, TBIs are accompanied by a brainstem injury and/or a coma. They also can be magnified, sometimes fatally, by secondary damage. A few other ways to describe a traumatic brain injury include diffuse axonal, acceleration/deceleration, coup contrecoup, and focal.

Finally, there are *acquired brain injuries* or *ABIs*, which cover those brain injuries that arise due to something other than trauma. Let's try to make some sense of this medical jargon, starting with the most common form of traumatic brain injury, closed head.

✗ Closed Head Injuries

The majority of traumatic brain injuries are closed head. The skull is left intact and the trauma to the brain is not visible. Closed head injuries usually occur when some form of trauma causes the head to rapidly switch direction. This propels the brain ricocheting back and forth against the sharp interior knobs of the skull bones, traumatizing tissue.

- Axons are pushed and pulled haphazardly, causing widespread devastation and upsetting millions of delicate nerve messages.
- Harmful chemicals can be released into the brain causing further damage.
- Arteries and veins within the brain can tear, leaking blood into the skull.
- This blood can form a pool (*hematoma*), which can push into the brain compressing tissue and squeezing neurons.
- Traumatized brain tissue bleeds and swells, creating pressure inside the inflexible skull. This is called *intracranial pressure* or *ICP*.
- Intracranial pressure can lead to *secondary damage*, which can be more harmful than the initial injury.

Open Head Injuries

In an open head traumatic brain injury, an external force tears open the scalp, cracks the skull, rips apart the membranes, and pierces the brain.

- Skull, skin, hair, and debris are jammed into the brain creating bruising, bleeding (*hemorrhage*), and swelling (*edema*).
- Umpteen neurons are destroyed.
- Gazillions of pathways among neurons are severed.
- The brain is exposed to the outside, inviting infection and further harm.
- If the skull was fractured or displaced, the injured portion of the brain has room to swell.

Brainstem Injury

In a brainstem injury, the bundles of nerves that control the body's automatic processes are twisted or torn as the brain caroms around the skull.

- Trauma to the brainstem can result in a characteristic type of paralysis of the arms and legs. The legs are stretched out straight and stiff, the arms bent up at the elbow.
- In graver brainstem injuries, limb movement is awkward and uncoordinated.
- Trauma to the brainstem can inhibit the body's automatic wake-up response, leaving the patient in a coma.
- If the brainstem is inactive, the patient has little hope of recovery.

41

Secondary Damage

Recovery from a brain injury does not start immediately after the initial trauma. Secondary—sometimes even fatal—damage can occur hours, days, or weeks later. In fact, this secondary damage, if not addressed, can be more harmful than the initial blow.

Secondary damage occurs when the bleeding and swelling of injured brain tissue crowd into the finite space of the rigid skull. This elevates the patient's intracranial pressure. As pressure rises within the skull, three life-threatening events can happen:

- Healthy brain tissue can be forced into the rough inner surface of the skull, causing more damage, more swelling, more bleeding, and even higher intracranial pressure.
- Healthy brain tissue can be squeezed and damaged.
- The brainstem can be jammed down into the vertebrae (*herniation*), triggering or prolonging a coma, and interfering with life-sustaining functions.

Other secondary dangers doctors watch for after a brain injury include:

- Obstructed breathing, which can deprive the brain of oxygen
- Blood loss, which can lower blood pressure and reduce the supply of blood and oxygen to the brain
- Seizures
- Extreme agitation, which can increase ICP
- The release of chemicals toxic to nerve cells
- Injuries to other organs and systems, which can complicate treatment of the brain injury

Trauma physicians have a number of options to stabilize the patient and limit secondary brain damage. They can:

- Attach the patient to a ventilator to ensure an adequate supply of oxygen and to keep her breathing should herniation occur.
- Monitor her blood pressure.
- Lower her body temperature to slow brain activity.
- Limit the fluids flowing into her body and to her brain.
- Implant an ICP monitor to measure her intracranial pressure.
- Restrict visits that can stimulate the patient and elevate her ICP.
- Perform surgery to drain excess fluid and/or remove destroyed tissue if the patient's ICP reaches critical levels.
- Administer medication to

  o Prevent further swelling
  o Calm an agitated patient
  o Neutralize and prevent the toxic effects of chemicals released in the brain
  o Prevent blood pressure from rising too high or falling too low

Diffuse Axonal Injury

An injury is labeled diffuse when multiple areas of the brain are involved. This typically occurs after a sudden *acceleration* or *deceleration* of the skull, as happens, for example, in a motor vehicle crash. When Jessica's car was struck by the rapidly traveling SUV, her body was held in place by her seat belt, but her brain was launched like a basketball, rebounding off the inside of her skull many times.

43

With a diffuse axonal injury, a vast number of neurons are twisted, stretched, and/or compressed. Since the damage occurs on a microscopic level, the devastation—though considerable—may not appear on *CT (computed tomography) scans*, the doctor's number one tool in detecting a brain injury.

Coup Contrecoup Injury

Another form of traumatic brain injury is the coup contrecoup injury, which causes a *cerebral contusion* or a bruise to the brain.

A coup injury occurs at the site of the brain that either slams into the skull when the head stops abruptly or absorbs the impact of an object, such as a brick wall or a baseball bat.

A contrecoup injury occurs when the force of the coup injury is strong enough to propel the brain to the opposite side of the skull. In this case, the brain is bruised in two areas.

Coup and contrecoup traumas are called *focal* injuries in which the harm is limited to one or two areas, as opposed to the widespread damage of an acceleration-deceleration diffuse axonal injury.

Acquired Brain Injury

Unlike traumatic brain injuries, which are triggered by an external force, acquired brain injuries result from some internal event, such as a stroke, heart attack, aneurysm, tumor, infection, disease, poisoning, or substance abuse that disrupts the normal operations of the brain's neurons.

Acquired brain injuries also occur when there is an interruption in the supply of blood and oxygen flowing to the brain. Without oxygen, neurons begin to die after about four minutes.

At our elementary level of discussion, the consequences of a brain injury—traumatic or acquired—for the survivor are similar.

Note: Recently, the definition of acquired brain injury has been broadened by some to include all damage to the brain acquired after birth, including traumatic injuries. Obviously, this can cause some confusion when using and interpreting this term.

The Healing Brain

The medical world has developed ways to keep people with horrendous brain injuries alive, but it has not yet found ways to return these patients to their pre-injury condition. The human brain has an amazing ability to heal itself, but once neurons are dead, they are gone for good. Once the connections among neurons are severed, they cannot be reattached. This is why all survivors of a serious brain injury suffer some permanent impairment.

This does not mean that people living with a brain injury cannot improve their condition. Nearly all survivors—through hard work—are able to regain some capabilities lost to their injuries.

How are they able to do this?

- The brain begins to heal once the patient's condition is stabilized.
- Injured brain tissue stops bleeding; swelling subsides.
- Surviving neurons reactivate.
- Damaged—not dead—neurons repair themselves.
- The brain rewires itself, growing new pathways among the billions of still healthy neurons.

- Through a process called plasticity, healthy portions of the brain assume some of the functions previously performed by the destroyed neurons.
- In rehabilitation, survivors relearn and practice lost skills until the instructions for performing these tasks are, once again, hardwired into their brain.
- Also, in rehabilitation, patients are taught to compensate for their deficits by learning new ways to perform activities impacted by their injury.

For maximum benefit, survivors should begin formal rehabilitation as soon as they are responding to commands. This enables professionally guided therapy to work in sync with the natural healing of the brain.

Recovering from a serious brain injury is a mammoth undertaking. In the initial days of their recovery, survivors often are as helpless as an infant. The connections among billions of neurons in their brain have been severed. Messages cannot pass. The activities dependent on these messages—even a task as simple as getting out of bed—are unmanageable.

Jessica complained of an aching leg whenever she lay on her left side. She endured this pain because she couldn't recall how to change her position in bed. For Jessica to once again be able to switch from her left side to her right side she had to relearn and practice this simple maneuver until she had mastered it.

Given that it takes a lifetime to accumulate the information stored in one's brain, it's not surprising that recovery can be a lifelong process. The brain is the slowest part of the human body to heal. The spontaneous recovery of damaged neurons takes months. The rewiring of the brain can take much longer.

5

The Litany of Uncertainty
It Will Be Months Before
We Know For Sure

The first day of our new life seemed endless. I made the phone calls no one ever wants to receive. "Jessica's been in a terrible car accident," I told family, friends, and coworkers. "She's in a coma; she may die." I had neither the time nor the energy to sugarcoat this news or comfort its recipients.

Our good friend Michael was the first of a steady stream of visitors to pass through the hospital that unhappy day. Soon after Michael's arrival, Dr. Thomas, the Chief of Trauma Services, paid his first visit. He was a tall, dignified gentleman, always impeccably outfitted in a spotless physician's white coat, a stethoscope dangling around his neck, moving around the hospital with the energy of a much younger man.

Dr. Thomas got right to the point.

"Your wife has a severe brain injury. Pressure is building inside her skull," he said. "If we can control the pressure, she'll make it. If not, we'll lose her."

After a tense moment, he continued, "I think she'll make it. We've had good luck with this type of injury."

I started breathing again.

"I expect the swelling and bleeding to peak in about forty-eight hours," he added. "We'll know much more then."

Dr. Thomas also reported damage to Jessica's brainstem, which had been twisted violently as her brain rattled around her skull in the collision. This, he explained, was why she was in a coma.

"I have every expectation her brainstem will heal and your wife will wake up," he said. "But she may not. This can be a very slow process."

He cautioned us to watch for improvement on a weekly, not a daily, basis. He tried to encourage us by saying he was pleased that her condition had not deteriorated since she arrived at the hospital.

After allowing time for these two bombshells to explode, Dr. Thomas had more painful news. This he delivered with certainty.

"With a trauma of this magnitude, the woman you knew this morning is gone," he said. "Only time will tell how much she'll be transformed by this injury."

We were silent for a minute. Then Michael broke the tension. "I hope she's not so bossy this time." We laughed, releasing some of our skyrocketing panic.

"I can't really say what the nature and extent of her impairments will be," Dr. Thomas continued. "They may completely change your lives or they may be inconsequential."

Looking back, those last three words—"may be inconsequential"—were wishful thinking. Given the extent of the trauma to Jessica's brain, it was certain she would suffer considerable impairment. I wonder whether Dr. Thomas's intent was to dispense the bad news slowly, giving me time to digest one bitter morsel at a time. Or, perhaps, his aim was to give me some cause to be hopeful in an otherwise bleak scenario.

With one foot out the door, Dr. Thomas listed Jessica's other injuries: broken hip and pelvic bones, bruised internal organs, and a collapsed lung. "Nothing dire that requires surgery, but her injuries are excruciating," he warned. "So she will be heavily sedated, which could extend her coma." Dr. Thomas assured us that these injuries would heal quickly and have minimal lasting effect. This was more wishful thinking. Jessica still is plagued by chronic nerve pain from her fractures.

(Months later, we learned that the trauma team overlooked a fracture to Jessica's right wrist. This is not unusual with a serious brain injury. A comatose patient can't point to where it hurts.)

I had umpteen questions about Jessica's brain injury and her prognosis, but Dr. Thomas had few answers. Before moving on to his other patients and their families, he recited a phrase or two from the Litany of Uncertainty, which would become more and more frustrating with each repetition.

Take it one day at a time.

Every brain injury is unique.

We'll just have to wait and see.

There's no substitute for waiting.

It will be months before we know for sure.

An hour later, as I was still agonizing over Dr. Thomas's grim report, Dr. Roberts approached with a welcome cold can of ginger ale and a pack of graham crackers. Her consideration momentarily consoled me.

Dr. Roberts was seeking my permission to include Jessica among 720 participants in a clinical trial of a new medication. I scanned the jargon-filled material describing the study. In my state of shock, I couldn't follow the papers I was being asked to sign.

Dr. Roberts assured me that Jessica's participation in the trial, "may help her, but definitely will not harm her." This guarantee sounded a bit one-sided to me, but I trusted that the downside was slight and well worth the potential benefit to future brain injury patients.

With not even a trace of coercion and exaggerated sensitivity, Dr. Roberts stressed the need for a quick answer. In light of Jessica's habitual willingness to help others, and with Michael's concurrence, it became an easy choice. I enrolled Jessica in the study. She and I are happy with this decision, though, we were unable to discover whether Jessica received the trial medication or if the study was a success.

The rest of the day passed in a blur: the phone calls, the all-too-brief visits with Jessica, the coming and going of relatives and friends, and my largely fruitless efforts to speak to a doctor. I'm a patient man. Jessica says I'm too patient. I wasn't asking for much, just two or three minutes with one of the slew of specialists dashing in and out of the intensive care unit.

The day's activities normally would have exhausted me. The adrenaline that shot through my body when I learned of the accident kept me going well into the afternoon.

I'm disabled by a largely untreatable condition currently called chronic myofascial pain. Every few years, the name changes as more research is conducted. My illness limits my ability to perform activities most people take for granted: writing, typing, operating a computer, just about any repetitive motion. At times, even turning the pages of a book or holding a newspaper is painful. I worried that my body wouldn't cope well with the physical and emotional rigors of supporting Jessica through her recovery.

Not surprisingly, late that afternoon my energy vanished, my optimism plummeted, and I was frantic with fear. The all-too-real possibility that I would lose Jessica—through death or infirmity—monopolized my thoughts. To no one in particular, I confessed, "I don't think Jessica's going to make it. I'm trying to prepare myself."

Jessica's youngest brother, Robert, who had just arrived, tried to lift my spirits. "Jessica's a strong woman," he said. "Let's stay positive here."

Jessica's father, Richard, added that Jessica was the first of his seven children to "get in my face if she disagreed with me. If anyone's tough enough to get through this, it's Jessica."

They claim that at that moment my attitude swung 180 degrees. I took control, sending Michael to the hospital library for a book on brain injury and assigning Robert and his wife Elizabeth the overnight shift with Jessica.

After this final burst of energy, the adrenaline was gone and I got a lift home. I intended to relax for an hour or so. I turned on music and lay down on the couch, but soon realized rest was impossible. My muscles ached and my mind was racing with a jumble of thoughts, ranging from the monumental "What will I do if Jessica dies?" to the mundane "When should I feed the cats?"

I put my nervous energy to work. I cleaned the refrigerator. As I purged, scrubbed, and rearranged, I was startled to recall that earlier in the day, I heard the sirens of rescue vehicles, never imagining they were coming for Jessica. Today, when I'm home and I hear sirens, I'm still reminded of Jessica's car crash.

Later that evening, I returned to the hospital. I had three minutes with Dr. Thomas, who, I realized a week later, never appeared to go home. He had nothing new to offer, just one or two lines from the Litany of Uncertainty.

As evening turned to darkness, my sister Barbara drove me home. I was exhausted, my nerves were frazzled, and in my discombobulated state I was useless to Jessica. A nurse expressed surprise and mild disapproval that I wasn't going to spend the night with Jessica. But it was painfully clear I would need to monitor my health constantly to be able to support Jessica in the taxing days, weeks, and months ahead.

Late that night Barbara and I frantically made plans for the next few days. We compiled lists of names and telephone numbers. We reviewed insurance policies. We sought and dove into any odd job, anything to postpone facing our fears. Barbara would be my anchor for the next month.

Before climbing into bed at midnight, I called the ICU. Jessica was still unconscious. She was totally unresponsive, even to the painful prick of a nurse's pin. I later learned that these are the characteristics of *Level 1: No Response* on the Rancho Los Amigos Scale of Cognitive Functioning.

To calm myself, I replayed the words of Dr. Thomas assuring me that survivors of serious brain injuries often enjoy full and satisfying—albeit transformed—lives after their rehabilitation. I simply told myself Jessica would be one of these successful survivors. This was a naïve approach, I knew, but I hoped it would give me the strength to climb out of bed the next morning.

I also was comforted by the memory that Jessica and I shared a hasty, but warm, goodbye that morning. If those were my last minutes with "my Jessica," I would remember them with love.

As I drifted to sleep, family, friends, and colleagues near and far were sending us positive energy. Some turned to prayer, relying on God's grace. Others sought a spiritual connection within a universal consciousness.

For the more mundane-minded—myself included—Jessica's survival hinged on a combination of factors: the randomness of the intersection of physics and human anatomy, the skills of her doctors and nurses, the miracles of modern medicine, and the good fortune to be within a brief ambulance ride to an excellent hospital.

6

Brain Injury Basics #2
Doctors, Comas, and Quantifying
Consciousness

One of my biggest mistakes during Jessica's hospitalization was passively waiting for her doctors to come to me. I was reluctant to summon them. Consequently, my numerous questions about Jessica's condition and prognosis often went unanswered for days at a time. I open this chapter with some suggestions for building mutually respectful and productive relationships with your survivor's doctors.

Also in this chapter, I introduce two important tools used by physicians to measure and describe the level of consciousness and behavior of brain injury patients: the Glasgow Coma Scale and the Rancho Los Amigos Scale of Cognitive Functioning. Next, I discuss what it means to be in a coma, exploding some popular myths. I also describe how readers should interact with their comatose family member. Finally, I discuss the easily confused terms persistent vegetative and minimally conscious states.

Dealing with Doctors

Doctors always seem to be in a rush. This is unfortunate for family and friends pacing in the intensive care waiting room, desperate for news about their survivor.

When seeking the attention of your doctors, be aware that there is a fine line between being assertive and being annoying. This fine line differs from doctor to doctor, day to day, patient to patient, and who knows what other variables.

I rarely approached this line. While I was always alert for opportunities to intercept one of Jessica's doctors entering or exiting the ICU, I dared not disturb them too frequently.

When doctors do provide you the opportunity to ask questions, they often respond with rapid-fire doses of medical jargon, which can be unintelligible and intimidating to the uninitiated. Medical terminology allows a busy doctor to pack a lot of information into a few words. Unfortunately, for most of us, they may as well be speaking Ukrainian.

The following suggestions, culled from my mistakes and the more productive experiences of the caregivers on the panel, will make your time with the doctors more fruitful and congenial.

- Be persistent, but polite. This advice may sound obvious, but after spending days in that pressure cooker known as the ICU waiting room, it's easy to lose your cool. You don't want your doctors dreading the time they spend with you.

- Don't always wait for the doctor to approach you. Expect and demand (nicely) a comprehensive briefing at least every two days. If your patient's condition is not yet stable, expect a full briefing every day.

- Don't expect or demand a briefing from the doctor more than once a day unless there's been a change in your patient's condition.

- Before calling the doctor, see if a nurse can handle your concern.

- Always watch for opportunities to speak with every doctor treating your loved one. This will give you multiple perspectives on your patient's condition. Physicians, such as an orthopedist or a neurologist, are more knowledgeable about certain areas of care. The first can tell you how well a broken bone will heal. The second can explain how your survivor may act as she emerges from her coma.

- Be well-prepared to speak with the doctor. Always have on hand a list of up-to-date questions to ask when opportunities arise. Arrange these questions in a logical order. Try to anticipate the answers so you're ready with thoughtful and probing follow-up questions.

- Ask for permission to tape record your conversations. Later, you can review the tape with others and learn more than you might have otherwise. Certain physicians, however, will object to this. Audio tapes can pop up in court.

- If you don't understand the doctor's responses, say so. You might say, "I'm having a hard time understanding what you just said. Please explain it again, using an example or simplifying your language."

- Be aware that there may not be an answer to some of your questions. Much is still unknown about the brain. Unfortunately, doctors don't have all the answers.

- Whenever possible, have someone join you for conversations with the doctor. This person can take notes, provide another perspective on the issues discussed, and help you digest the information later.

- Ask about alternatives to the treatments the doctor has chosen. Playing out alternative treatment scenarios is an appropriate topic of discussion between physician and family.

- Ask for a second opinion or a referral if you're concerned about the treatment plan for your patient or if you have doubts about the doctor's familiarity with brain injury. Brain injuries are complex and require specialized expert medical treatment, which is not available in many hospitals.

- If privacy regulations are barring the doctor from speaking to you, consider filing for a limited guardianship with the Clerk of the Courts (see the blue pages of your phone book). Thanks to the Health Insurance Portability and Accountability Act (HIPPA), hospitals strictly enforce privacy policies.

As you follow these recommendations, certain doctors will be miffed that you're consuming so much of their time. Most, however, will appreciate your efforts to understand what's happening to your survivor. They may even sit down with you for a few minutes.

The Glasgow Coma Scale

The Glasgow Coma Scale (GCS) is a universally applied measure of the severity of a brain injury. It is calculated either at the scene of the injury or in the emergency room. The GCS also is used with patients who remain unconscious for days, weeks, or months to gauge the depth of their coma and to assess whether they are improving or deteriorating.

The GCS assigns a numerical value to the patient's reaction to an attention-grabbing event, such as a prick with a pin or a shouted command, in three areas: eye opening, body movement, and speech. To calculate a GCS score add the numbers from each of these three areas, as indicated below, to obtain a figure which varies from three (the worst response) to fifteen (the best response).

Eye Opening

Opens eyes spontaneously	4
Opens eyes to speech	3
Opens eyes to pain	2
Does not open eyes	1

Body Movement

Obeys simple commands	6
Attempts to move from pain	5
Withdraws from pain	4
Moves muscles abnormally	3
Moves muscles involuntarily	2
Does not respond to pain	1

Speech

Speaks clearly and appropriately	5
Converses with confusion	4
Uses inappropriate words	3
Makes incomprehensible sounds	2
Makes no sounds	1

Eye Opening + Body Movement + Speech
= Glasgow Coma Scale Score

13 – 15	Mild Brain Injury
9 – 12	Moderate Brain Injury
3 – 8	Severe Brain Injury

Warning: The GCS is a broad measure of how well patients will recover. Its predictive value for any single individual—your survivor, for example—is suspect. Predicting the long-term outcome of a brain injury is riskier than roulette.

Some doctors don't share GCS scores with the family, particularly if the score is low. They argue that the additional bad news of a low GCS score heightens the family's anguish without providing any useful information.

But the old-school physicians of the past—"Let me worry about the numbers, little lady"—have been overtaken by the information age. Don't be surprised if your computer-savvy teenager greets you at home asking, "What's Mom's GCS?"

Remember, every brain injury is unique and unpredictable. Not everyone with a low GCS score has a bad outcome. Not everyone with a high GCS score has a good outcome. Many factors determine how well a person recovers from a brain injury. (See page 101.)

Many survivors on the panel had low GCS scores and yet today are leading productive lives. They include full-time high school and college students, volunteers in the community, an auto mechanic, a certified nurse's assistant, an attorney, a part-time management consultant, and a college professor.

This group also includes mothers and fathers, sons and daughters, and husbands and wives who relish each day, enjoy loving relationships, and bring joy to those around them.

The Glasgow Coma Scale is just one tool in a doctor's medical bag and just one more piece of information you can use to better comprehend your survivor's condition.

What Is a Coma?

A coma is a state of deep unconsciousness in which the patient is:

- Unaware of her surroundings
- Cannot be awakened
- Does not respond normally to stimuli, such as pain, sound, and light
- Performs no purposeful acts, such as opening her eyes or lifting her arm in response to a command

The common perception of a comatose person is someone who lies motionless with her eyes closed. This is just the first stage of a coma. In later stages, the patient can be hyperactive, moving her eyes back and forth, uttering sounds or even words, and performing what appear to be *purposeful acts*. These seemingly intentional movements, however, are *involuntary neurological responses* that the body performs automatically in response to internal needs or changes in the external environment.

Many survivors fall into a coma immediately after the blow to their brain. This occurs for one of two reasons: the neural pathways of the brain are critically disrupted or nerves in the brainstem are torn. Occasionally, a doctor will induce a coma to control the swelling of damaged brain tissue to prevent the potentially catastrophic consequences of soaring intracranial pressure.

The length of a coma varies with the seriousness of the injury. A coma can last minutes, hours, days, weeks, or, rarely, months or years. Physicians are unable to predict when a person will awake from a coma. No scientifically proven treatment for arousing a comatose patient has been found. The brain and the brainstem heal on their own timetable.

While in a coma, the patient must be safeguarded from the potentially debilitating consequences of being bed-ridden for a prolonged period. These precautions include:

- Providing nutrition through a tube threaded through the patient's nose (a *Nasogastric* or *NG tube*) or a tube inserted directly into her stomach (a *Gastric* or *G tube*)
- Rotating her body to prevent bedsores
- Moving her limbs through range of motion exercises and splinting her arms and/or legs to prevent *spasticity*, *contractures*, or muscle loss
- Positioning her upright in bed or sitting her in a chair
- Protecting her from infections, especially pneumonia

In the movies, people snap out of a coma as though a light switch had been flipped. One moment they are unconscious, the next, they're chowing down dinner. In the real world, emerging from a coma is akin to the gradual brightening of a room with a super-sensitive dimmer switch. The return to full consciousness is nearly always a gradual, mostly imperceptible process of increasing awareness and responsiveness.

A patient is considered no longer comatose when she is performing purposeful acts, such as responding appropriately to commands, like "Raise your arm" or "Squeeze my hand."

Other movements, such as the patient turning her head in the direction of voices or trying to remove her hand from a tight splint, are possible, perhaps even likely, but not clear, signs of arousal.

Family members, who spend many hours with the patient, often are delighted prematurely by twitches or gestures and other involuntary neurological responses. They also, however, are likely to be the first to witness the purposeful acts of an awakening patient. Doctors, though, often distrust the validity of observations made by hopeful family members.

Stimulating a Comatose Patient

We don't know whether the efforts of the family to rouse a patient from a coma actually work. It's impossible to know what a person in a coma experiences. Any memories she may have afterward are suspect because the operations of her brain are in such disarray it's difficult to separate a conscious memory from a subconscious dream. Many caregivers on the panel, however, are certain that their efforts were pivotal to their survivor's awakening.

Before stimulating your comatose survivor, discuss your plans with the doctors and nurses. If intracranial pressure is a concern, your interactions should be strictly limited. Stimulation of any kind can elevate ICP and endanger the patient's life. Otherwise, most physicians won't object to the following guidelines. Don't be surprised, however, if your doctor responds, "You can do whatever you want, but it won't make any difference."

- Use your regular tone of voice.
- Identify yourself each time you approach the patient.
- Assume she can hear and understand everything you say.
- Talk to her as if she were awake and able to understand you.
- Never discuss her progress, her lack of progress, or your personal fears in her presence.
- Keep it simple; too much stimulation can puzzle and agitate the patient.
- Tell her she has been injured and is in the hospital.
- Reassure her that she's being well cared for.
- Touch and gently stroke her; hold her hand.
- Talk about everyday things that will interest her.
- Surround her with familiar objects: photos, posters, toys, and mementos.
- Play her favorite music.
- Tape a soothing message that can be played when you're away.
- Don't ask questions. Instead of asking, "Do you know who I am;" say "I'm your husband, Garry."
- Play her favorite television shows and movies.
- Bring in companion animals (with permission from the nurses).
- Avoid constant stimulation; comatose patients need their rest.

Be creative. Use a wide variety of stimulants, such as bells, aromatherapy candles, cinnamon on the lips, and gentle massage. One caregiver on the panel played a tape of the sounds made by her husband's tools—his drill, buzz saw, and staple gun. Another played music her son despised, hoping to provoke a reaction. A third climbed into bed with her husband and held him tenderly. Be cautious and discuss your plans with the doctors and nurses.

There are formal—but controversial—coma arousal therapies in which multiple stimuli, usually packaged as coma stimulation kits, are presented to the patient in a systematic manner. These therapies have benefits. They give the family an active role in the treatment of their survivor, relieving some of their helplessness. Also, they may shorten the coma.

Coma arousal therapy, however, can be time consuming, expensive, and may raise false hopes. It also may prolong a coma through excessive stimulation. The jury is still out on the effectiveness of coma arousal therapy.

Vegetative and Minimally Conscious States

A coma usually does not persist for more than three or four weeks, and rarely for more than a few months. After this period, the patient may be considered to be in a "vegetative state." However, there is no clear delineation between "coma" and "vegetative state." As more time passes, the term "persistent vegetative state" may be used. Only a very small percentage of brain injury survivors remain in a persistent vegetative state.

A patient in a persistent vegetative state remains unaware of her environment. She may track moving objects with her eyes, experience sleep/wake cycles, shed tears, swallow, vocalize, and respond reflexively or automatically to sounds, touch, or pain. She also will perform all of her body's vegetative functions, such as heart rate and rhythm, digestion, and respiration. However, she still does not respond appropriately to commands. If this condition persists for more than one year, the patient may be said to be in a "permanent vegetative state."

When a patient is beginning to show signs of emerging from a coma or a vegetative state, she may be said to be in a "minimally conscious state" in which there is minimal, but definite, behavioral evidence of an emerging self-consciousness and/or awareness of the environment.

These terms are not clearly defined and they often are misunderstood by the general public. Whether your survivor is in a deep coma, a vegetative state, a light coma, or a minimally conscious state is far less important than the more concrete distinction between someone who does or does not respond appropriately to commands.

The Rancho Los Amigos Scale

For caregivers desperate for something solid to hold on to, the Rancho Los Amigos Scale of Cognitive Functioning is an oasis in a desert of uncertainty. As one caregiver on the panel told me, "Watching my husband move up the Rancho Scale helped me keep my sanity."

The Rancho Scale is a tool widely used to classify and track a patient's degree of functioning. This mostly objective scale begins at *Level 1*, when the patient is in a deep coma. It ends with *Level 10*[1], when the patient is acting independently, purposefully, and appropriately.

Warning: Graduating to *Level 10* does not mean the patient has returned to her pre-injury condition. Serious brain injuries always leave indelible marks on those who survive them.

The Rancho Scale also is used to determine when a person is able to benefit from rehabilitation. Some rehab facilities require patients to be at *Levels 3 or 4* before admitting them. Certain health insurers will not pay for rehabilitation until the patient has advanced to *Levels 3 or 4*.

Typically, the family, who spends much more time with the patient, detects progress to the next Rancho level well before the doctors. This can be maddening if you are waiting, as I was, for your survivor to be declared ready for rehab by her doctor.

---

[1] Note: The Rancho Scale originally had eight levels. In 1998, the third edition of the scale was expanded to include Levels 9 and 10. Some medical professionals and facilities still use the eight-level scale.

Rancho Los Amigos Scale of Cognitive Functioning

Level 1: No Response. The patient is unconscious. She does not react to attempts to stimulate a response, such as a painful prick with a pin or a shouted command. She can be in this condition for hours, days, weeks or, rarely, months or years.

Level 2: Generalized Response. The patient reacts inconsistently and without purpose to stimuli. Her initial response is triggered, most often, by deep pain. This response, often a reflexive body movement or a garbled vocalization, usually is the same regardless of the stimulus.

Level 3: Localized Response. The patient reacts more appropriately, but still inconsistently, to stimuli, especially bright light, sound, and physical discomfort. She inconsistently follows simple commands, such as "Close your eyes" or "Squeeze my hand." She may occasionally turn her head in the direction of a speaker's voice.

Level 4: Confused-Agitated. The patient is alert and restless. She's confused because she doesn't understand what's happened to her. Her attention span is short. Her behavior is without purpose and can be bizarre. She may cry out or try to remove her feeding tube. She can be hostile and uncooperative.

Level 5: Confused-Inappropriate. The patient has developed a broad interest in her surroundings. She still responds to simple commands without purpose. She is easily distracted and needs frequent reminders to stay on task. If overstimulated, she becomes agitated. She doesn't initiate activities and is unable to absorb new information. Her social interactions are inappropriate. She responds mostly to pain and close family and friends.

Level 6: Confused-Appropriate. The patient now is motivated, but she still depends on others to lead the way. Her reactions are more appropriate. If uncomfortable, she complains. She easily follows simple directions and is beginning to recognize her therapists. She is more aware of herself and her family and friends. Her orientation to time and place is inconsistent. Her memory of the past has improved, but her memory of recent events is still shaky.

Level 7: Automatic-Appropriate. The patient acts appropriately in the hospital and at home, but her skills deteriorate in unfamiliar environments. She goes about her daily routine robotically. Although she can dress, wash, and feed herself independently, she needs super-vision to ensure her safety. Her judgment and problem-solving skills are still impaired. She cannot make realistic plans for the future.

Level 8: Purposeful-Appropriate-Standby Assistance. The patient is alert and consistently oriented to person, place, and time. She is independent and functional at home and in the community. However, she has subtle problems with self-evaluation, reasoning, information processing, and judgment, especially in unusual situations. She uses memory devices, such as calendars, notes, and timers, to compensate for her poor memory. She can be irritable, easily frustrated, and self-centered.

Level 9: Purposeful-Appropriate-Standby Assistance on Request. The patient now is aware of her impairments and has learned to compensate for them. She is able to complete and shift between familiar tasks independently. With standby assistance, she uses assistive memory devices to recall her schedule. She anticipates problems and is concerned that her social behavior be appropriate.

Level 10: Purposeful-Appropriate-Modified Independent. The patient can multi-task. She initiates and completes unfamiliar tasks that may require compensatory strategies. She understands how her impairments impact her behavior. She weighs the consequences of her decisions. Her social interactions are consistently appropriate.

Warning: Recovery from a brain injury rarely is as simple and straightforward as the Rancho Scale suggests. Some patients zoom through the Rancho levels. Some improve and then regress to a lower level before advancing again. Some plateau at a certain level. Remember, every brain injury is unique and unpredictable.

Checklist for Success #1
The First Few Days

___ Do you know that it's best to look for improvement in your survivor's condition on a weekly, rather than a daily, basis?

___ Do you understand that in the early days of a brain injury it is impossible to predict the nature and extent of the impairments your survivor will suffer?

___ Have you begun a journal that includes:

- A brief medical history and list of medications taken by your survivor prior to the brain injury
- The name, specialty, and telephone number of the doctors treating your survivor
- The doctors' treatment plans and goals for your survivor
- Your impression of your survivor's condition
- Any changes you see in your survivor's condition
- All instructions you receive from the doctors and nurses
- Your observations on the care your survivor is receiving

___ Are you wondering how best to interact with your survivor's doctors? If so, see page 54.

___ Have you prepared a list of questions to ask the doctors? Don't forget to update this list regularly.

___ Have you established guidelines for visitors? You
should:

- Decide beforehand who may visit your survivor.
- Prepare visitors for what they will see, especially if
your survivor has an ICP monitor.
- Expect relatives and friends to react and cope
differently.
- Insist that visitors remain positive.

___ Are you familiar with the Glasgow Coma Scale (GCS)?
What was your survivor's GCS score when she arrived
at the hospital? [See page 57.]

___ What do you know about comas?

- Comatose individuals do not always lie quietly;
they can be hyperactive.
- People do not snap out of a coma? It is a very slow
process.
- How should you interact with a comatose person?
[See page 61.]

___ Do you recognize the difference between involuntary
neurological responses and the purposeful acts that
signal the end of a coma? [See page 59.]

___ Are you familiar with the Rancho Los Amigos Scale of
Cognitive Functioning? At what level is your survivor?
[See page 64.]

___ Do you know that you probably will see improvements
in your survivor s condition before the doctors?

____   Have you sought the support of those who know brain injury well? Here are some places to start:

- Brain Injury Association of America

    o (800) 444-6443
    o www.biausa.org
    o info@biausa.org

- Your state brain injury association

    o Ask about local support groups and peer mentors.
    o (800) 444-6443
    o www.biausa.org/stateoffices.htm
    o See page 234.

- Internet support groups

    o www.tbinet.org
    o www.tbihome.org
    o www.48friend.org
    o www.dailystrength.org
    o http://groups.yahoo.com
    o www.braininjurychat.org
    o www.avbi.org

____   Do you know that survivors of a serious brain injury often enjoy full and satisfying—albeit transformed—lives after their rehabilitation? It is important to remember this.

7

A Tsunami of Emotions
Two Lives Will Be Rearranged

When I awoke the day after Jessica's accident, I didn't immediately recall the events of the previous day. Then, as if hearing the news for the first time, I remembered the phone call, the rush to the ER, the horrifying accident scene, Jessica's motionless body, and the congregation of concerned family and friends at the hospital.

I was slammed by a tsunami of emotions: shock, panic, grief, and helplessness. I sobbed uncontrollably as I would for many mornings to come, releasing just enough of my feelings to gather myself, grab a piece of toast or two, drive my rented car to the hospital, and take my seat next to Jessica.

Unlike her first day in the ICU, when Jessica lay motionless in bed, she now occasionally slipped out of her tranquility. She opened her eyes wide, but they were unfocused, revealing no self-awareness. She scowled in response to the pain caused by her broken bones and battered internal organs. She flailed her arms and legs in an unconscious effort to shake off the life-preserving paraphernalia covering much of her body.

This new behavior indicated that Jessica had advanced to *Level 2: Generalized Response* on the Rancho Scale:

> **Level 2: Generalized Response.** The patient reacts inconsistently and without purpose to stimuli. Her initial response is triggered most often by deep pain. This response, often a reflexive body movement or a garbled vocalization, usually is the same regardless of the stimulus.

The good news—Jessica was improving—was tempered by a continuing danger. Whenever she became agitated or overstimulated, her intracranial pressure spiked. So, our visits with her were strictly limited. I was the only one permitted to speak to her. Others were instructed to identify themselves softly and hold her hand quietly for no more than a few minutes.

The days passed slowly. Our private waiting room, furnished with just a small couch, three chairs, and an end table often overflowed with people. Jessica's family alone filled it beyond capacity.

The coming and going of family and friends soon turned into a steady blur of faces, hugs, and words of encouragement. I automatically greeted each visitor and reported the same update on Jessica's condition without much thought or outward emotion, while that painful knot of panic and grief in my gut screamed for attention.

I discovered that certain folks, despite their unquestioned affection for Jessica, were too distraught to sit with her. I respected their feelings and was not disappointed by their squeamishness. The bolt protruding from Jessica's forehead was enough to discomfort most visitors.

At night, when Jessica was receiving much less stimulation from the medical staff, the nurses permitted more frequent visits. Jessica's sister, Laura, joined Robert and Elizabeth in their overnight vigil.

They spoke to Jessica softly about past shared adventures and their everyday lives, always watching the flashing numbers displayed on the ICP monitor screen. Robert had a knack for raising these numbers to dangerous levels and he often was shushed or sent back to the waiting room by the nurses.

As they passed the time, Jessica's siblings started recording their thoughts and observations—as well as messages of encouragement—in a journal they kept next to her bed. This became an easy way to keep her many visitors up to date on her progress. It also left me with an excellent multi-perspective account of Jessica's recovery, which I consulted frequently in writing this book.

When forty-eight hours passed with no deterioration in Jessica's condition, her prognosis improved considerably. She had suffered no significant loss of oxygen to her brain. The bleeding and swelling within her skull had subsided. Her intracranial pressure was under control.

"Jessica's not entirely out of the woods," Dr. Thomas told us. "But this is no longer a life-or-death situation."

When I asked him about Jessica's long-term prognosis, he remained more than cautious. "She will leave the hospital, but in what shape, we can't tell yet," was all Dr. Thomas was willing to say.

He warned us again that, undoubtedly, Jessica would have permanent brain damage. He encouraged us by suggesting that her impairments might be imperceptible. "She may even be able to resume her career," he offered.

This surprised me. I couldn't recall telling Dr. Thomas about the complexity and stress of Jessica's work. He probably saw a dejected spouse in need of a boost. Satisfying the families of brain injury patients must be one of the more challenging duties of a trauma physician.

Still hanging over our heads was the harrowing possibility that Jessica might not emerge from her coma. If the trauma to her brainstem was extensive, she wouldn't wake up. Dr. Thomas predicted that "in all probability" her "wakeup response" would be restored. Nonetheless, I knew that each additional day spent in a coma meant that Jessica's recovery would be more challenging.

Jessica still required assistance to breathe. She was attached to a ventilator and would remain so until her mental and neurological status improved. While connected to the ventilator, Jessica was vulnerable to a lethal form of pneumonia, which was developing a resistance to antibiotics.

A final concern—trivial compared to the others, but still a worry to me—was the long list of phone calls waiting to be made. Jessica is a warm, generous, and outgoing person. She has a large, scattered family and a wide circle of friends.

These were not quick and easy calls. Everyone I spoke to needed time to absorb the bad news. After the initial shock, they had questions, but I was pressed for time. I had to move quickly to the next call. Also, the introvert in me was reluctant to spend too much energy on the phone. Soon, just the sight of a telephone exhausted me.

To worsen matters, people kept calling the house for updates on Jessica's condition, to comfort me, and to be comforted in return. Comforting others, however, is not one of my strengths.

To maintain my sanity, I simply chose to ignore the ringing telephone and to quit returning messages. The tape in our answering machine filled up. The pile of unanswered messages taken by house guests spilled onto the floor. But each morning, I was up and off to the hospital, refreshed as much as possible, ready to face the formidable world of brain injury.

I didn't entirely abandon family and friends. Once a week, after dinner, I composed an email describing Jessica's condition.

I also used these messages to ask for help. I knew that supporting Jessica through her recovery and rehabilitation would be much too large a job for just one person, especially one with my disabilities. For Jessica's recovery to succeed, we would need lots of help, for months.

We kept a twenty-four-hour vigil throughout Jessica's week in the ICU, eagerly watching for signs she was waking. We first found hope when she opened her eyes. Dr. Thomas quickly squelched our excitement by explaining that eye opening amounted to only a one percent improvement in her condition. But it was improvement, we told ourselves.

Other events lifted our spirits. Jessica's movements at times looked to be the reawakening of self-awareness. She twirled her right foot and hand as though she were an infant discovering an exciting new skill. Laura, the optimist among us, was certain Jessica was doing this consciously, letting us know that everything will be all right.

At times, I imagined Jessica was trying to speak to me. "What happened? Where am I? I hurt. I'm scared." These thoughts always triggered in me an overwhelming sadness. I felt powerless to comfort Jessica. I stroked her arms and held her hand. I told her she was being well cared for. I said I missed her terribly, and assured her that she was improving every day, even when I feared otherwise.

Three days after Jessica's accident, my sister Barbara and I met with Tom, the ICU social worker. The meeting was a sobering reality check.

Tom, speaking with the certainty Dr. Thomas avoided, warned us that Jessica would not be able to return to work for at least a year, if ever. He recommended that we apply immediately for Social Security Disability Income since the process takes forever. Tom also advised us to study the fine print in Jessica's insurance policies. He suggested we may want to hire an attorney or a case manager to be certain Jessica obtained all of her entitled benefits.

Tom instructed us to start thinking about which rehabilitation facility we would use for the next step in Jessica's recovery. He cautioned us that rehabilitation is very expensive. Health insurance, he said, rarely covered the full cost of therapy. "It's not unusual for a family to be bankrupted by this," he said.

Finally, we had to appreciate how little control we had over Jessica's recovery. "It's a lengthy and complicated process. It will unfold in its own time," Tom explained. "But you can rely on Dr. Thomas. He's the best and he has a great interest in brain injury."

The next day, we had a thirty-minute briefing from Dr. Franklin, the second-in-command. As he entered our tiny haven just outside the ICU, Dr. Franklin was surprised by an audience of one shaken husband, surrounded by five energetic women armed with pens and notepads, ready to pepper him with questions. Jessica and I are friends with a fair number of bright, resourceful, self-confident, and outspoken women. My mother might call them unladylike, which they surely would take as a compliment.

Dr. Franklin opened with the bad news.

"The latest CT scan," he reported, "shows that Jessica's injury is more critical than we initially thought. Jessica has a severe brain injury and we can't predict the outcome," he said. "She'll probably do okay. We can't be certain for at least six months, maybe a year. She's stable; that should please you."

Dr. Franklin was concerned that Jessica was still at *Level 2* on the Rancho Scale. "I had hoped that after four days she'd be more responsive," he added. "She's totally unaware of her environment. She isn't responding to commands at all. Those movements you keep getting excited about are just involuntary neurological responses. They don't indicate any progress."

Dr. Franklin cautioned us to not hope for any dramatic headway in Jessica's condition. "The human brain has the flexibility to repair itself and to transfer certain functions from damaged to healthy areas. But this takes time." He urged us to be relieved that her condition hadn't worsened.

Most of all, he warned us against expecting a scene like those in the movies when the comatose patient pops up and asks, "What's for dinner?" In the real world, he explained, "When a person emerges from a coma, awareness returns gradually and is often accompanied by utter disorientation."

Dr. Franklin explained that he and Dr. Thomas had their own ways of viewing brain injuries. We might hear conflicting statements from them. "When this happens," he assured us, "don't be alarmed. We speak to each other throughout the day and always resolve our differences to each other's satisfaction."

Dr. Franklin then listed the positives. Jessica's condition was stable. The pressure within her skull was normal and they would soon remove the ICP monitor. Her body was absorbing the liquid nutrition pumped through her NG tube. Her internal bleeding had stopped, and her blood pressure was normal.

"Overall, Jessica's making progress," Dr. Franklin concluded, "She'll probably do well in her recovery."

Despite this good news, there was no ignoring the fact that Jessica would suffer some lifelong impairment. I replayed Dr. Thomas's words that Jessica would wake up a different person. What did he mean by that? In what ways will Jessica be altered? Will she lose those qualities that underlie the essence of her being? Will she be a new person, altogether? If so, will I be able to love this new person? Will this new person be able to love me? I found it best not to dwell on the more chilling possibilities.

Naïvely, I thought we'd have a comprehensive briefing on Jessica's condition every few days; we didn't. Our session with Dr. Franklin was our first and last opportunity to discuss Jessica's condition in detail. The ICU nurses told us that they always try to have at least one doctor meet with their patients' families each day. Sometimes they succeed; sometimes they fail.

So, we patiently waited. We watched for the tiniest changes in Jessica's condition and we hoped our worst fears would not be realized.

Notes

8

How to Succeed as a Caregiver
Focus on What
You Can Control

While you are unable to predict how well your survivor is going to recover, there are two things you can say with certainty: (1) she is facing the challenge of her life, and (2) she will need your undying support to succeed.

When your patient emerges from her coma, she will need you to comfort her through her bewilderment and agitation. In rehabilitation, she will need your encouragement as she is pushed to the limits of her ability. When she returns home, she will need your support in countless ways. Through all this, your loved one will rely on your patience, guidance, creativity, stamina, selflessness, and love. In other words, your survivor is going to demand every minute and every ounce of energy you can muster for a long time. It is now time to get ready for this demanding job.

This chapter is devoted to helping you prepare—physically, intellectually, emotionally, and spiritually—to be an excellent caregiver. It also reminds you that even the best caregivers require some help. I describe the Family and Medical Leave Act, which may allow you to stop working for a while, and I discuss the benefits of hiring a brain injury case manager. Finally, I close this lengthy chapter with a discussion of the variables that impact how well an individual recovers from a brain injury.

Take Care of Yourself

Studies show that caring for a person with a brain injury leaves you vulnerable to stress-related illnesses. So, how do you prepare yourself for this difficult job?

Let's start with your physical health. It's okay to skimp on sleep, munch on fast food, and ignore your exercise routine for a week or two. However, when the adrenalin and the nervous energy that have been keeping you going well beyond your normal limits fade, your survivor may be emerging from her coma or just starting her rehabilitation. This is not the time to run out of gas. So, follow Mom's advice:

- Get enough sleep.
- Eat well.
- Exercise.
- Have some fun.

Maybe Mom didn't mention that last one, but it's as crucial as the first three. I can't overstate the importance of taking occasional vacations from the unrelenting responsibilities of caregiving. I waited too long to refresh myself. At times, I was merely a presence, rather than a participant, in Jessica's care, and she suffered because of this.

Be kind to yourself. Take regular breaks from brain injury.

- Read a book about something other than brain injury.
- Go to a movie, a concert, a museum, or a sporting event.
- Take a walk. Go for a run.
- Knit a scarf. Play a round of golf. Sing a song.
- Find ways to relax. Meditate. Pray. Practice yoga.
- Stay in contact with family, friends, and colleagues.
- Talk about something other than brain injury.
- Laugh as often as you can.

Next, ask yourself what you know about brain injury. If you're like I was, the answer is probably "not much." So, resolve to learn as much as you can.

Reading this book is a wise first step. Then, if one family guide is not enough, here are two others that merit your attention:

- *Mindstorms: The Complete Guide for Families Living with Traumatic Brain Injury* by John W. Cassidy, M.D. with Karla Dougherty, Da Capo Press, 2009.
- *Head Injury: The Facts* by Audrey Daisley, Rachel Tams, and Udo Kischka, Oxford University Press, 2009.

Here are five other easy ways to learn more about brain injury:

1. Contact the Brain Injury Association of America (800-444-6443 & www.biausa.org) and/or your state brain injury association (see page 234). These organizations have an abundance of useful information, particularly on local resources.

2. Read the engaging and informative books described in the List of Essential Resources on pages 232 and 233. These include family guides, personal stories written by survivors and caregivers, and technical works authored by medical professionals.

3. Visit the excellent Web sites listed on pages 229 to 232.

4. Join a support group, either locally—ask the people at your state association—or online. Support groups are a great way to learn from the folks who have been there. They can give you valuable advice and guide you through the endless waves of emotions you're struggling to control. You also may find a new friend who knows exactly what you're going through. (See page 231.)

5. Keep an up-to-date list of questions for the doctors and don't hesitate to ask them every chance you get.

Now let's talk about how you're going to find the time to:

- Be a full-time caregiver to your survivor.
- Meet your obligations to family, job, studies, and the other demands of your life.
- Learn about brain injury.
- Have some fun.

Simply put, you're not. There aren't enough hours in the day.

If you haven't already been asking for help, start now. You shouldn't be spending twenty-four, or even twelve, hours a day at the hospital or rehabilitation facility. For some advice on asking for help, see page 92.

An Exception: Three panel members asked me to make an exception to this advice for mothers. As one told me, "I needed to be there every minute. It was just that simple."

Okay, I'll make an exception for moms, with one condition. Always remember that when your child comes home, even if she is an adult, she will be totally dependent on you, twenty-four hours a day, every day. If you compromise on your health now, you may be endangering her well-being later. At the first sign of declining health, please, take a break to refresh yourself.

Not only must you be physically fit to be an excellent caregiver, you also must be emotionally fit. You may not realize that emotions run amok can overwhelm and immobilize you. Caring for someone who has just acquired a brain injury leaves you vulnerable to at least ten emotions that can compromise your caregiving abilities.

	Shock	**Denial**	**Panic**	
Anger	**Guilt**	**Grief**	**Helplessness**
	Loneliness	**Fear**	**Depression**	

Just being aware of the potential havoc these emotions can wreak gives you a head start in handling them well.

Shock: This is a common reaction to any terrible news.

This can't be happening. It doesn't feel real.

Denial: Shock often leads to denial.

There must be a mistake. Jessica wouldn't drive like that.

Not my son. He'll be back to his old self in no time.

Shock and denial are healthy. They give you time to accept the reality of a sudden tragic event. They become unhealthy when allowed to linger. For example, too many survivors and caregivers deny that a serious brain injury is forever. Denial then becomes an insurmountable obstacle to a successful recovery.

Panic: Panic usually accompanies shock and denial. Your thoughts are jumbled. Your body is shaking. Adrenaline is shooting through your veins, making you restless, if not hyperactive. Nothing makes sense. You don't understand and you cannot recall what the physicians are saying. You're in no condition to make vital decisions.

On day two of Jessica's recovery, I asked Dr. Zimmerman— the neurosurgeon consulting on Jessica's case—the same question five times, never absorbing his response. Fortunately, Barbara was with me and she took over the questioning when Dr. Zimmerman lost his patience.

Shock, denial, and panic usually are short-term emotions. When they are preventing you from facing your survivor's injury realistically and rationally, it's best to have someone at your side to help you cope with the situation.

When the adrenaline stops flowing and you've had time to digest the bad news, other emotions can distract you from your caregiving responsibilities.

Anger: Something immensely unfair has happened to your survivor, to your family, and to you. Your lives are about to be changed dramatically. The future suddenly has become very cloudy. It's not unreasonable to be angry at:

- Your survivor, for putting herself at risk
- The person who caused the injury through recklessness
- Yourself, for somehow not preventing the injury

If you're really losing your cool, you may direct your anger at:

- The doctors for not being more definitive in their statements
- The nurses for not treating your patient better
- The custodian who mops the floor at an inconvenient time

Here are three suggestions for harnessing your anger:

1. Try to forgive everyone responsible for the injury—including the survivor and yourself. Blaming others accomplishes nothing. If you can't forgive, set blame aside for a while.

2. Vent your anger. Letting it boil will make you even angrier until you explode.

3. But be careful how you vent. Directing your anger at the people caring for your loved one—doctors, nurses, therapists, and health insurance bureaucrats, for example—is never beneficial and can be harmful.

Twice, in the early days of Jessica's recovery, I let anger overwhelm me. The first time I punched the wall of an elevator. The second time I screamed at Jessica's Uncle Elliot. No harm done. My weak punch didn't send me to the emergency room and Elliot understood my need to vent. A punching bag, however, would have been a better choice in the first case.

Guilt: Guilt is another potentially harmful emotion. Spending hours wondering what you could or should have done to prevent the injury will not help your patient recover. Don't lose sleep over the "why" questions.

Why did I let her drive at night? She's too young.

Why did I let him get a motorcycle? They're so dangerous.

There are no answers to these questions. Focus on the future, not the past. Accidents happen.

Guilt also can arise from how you have chosen to spread your time among your survivor, family, employer, and anyone else who depends on you. Remember, you can't satisfy everyone. You have made an informed decision regarding what's best for you, your patient, and others. Now, you mustn't allow guilt to weaken your resolve to stick to that decision.

Guilt can be unhealthy in two ways:

1. It can crowd out the positive emotions—joy, hope, and determination—essential to being an excellent caregiver.
2. It can cause you to try to absolve yourself by attempting to be a superhuman caregiver.

Grief: Grief is a natural and healthy response to a brain injury. You, too, are a victim. But, unlike death and a funeral, there's no social convention for publicly acknowledging your grief. Most people are ignorant of the life-altering consequences of a brain injury. You may not receive the support you need to work your way through the mourning process.

Coping with your grief is a crucial aspect of your recovery. Here are six suggestions for healthy grieving:

1. Don't allow yourself to be rushed. Everyone grieves at his own pace.
2. The only way to get past your grief is to experience it.
3. Let it ebb slowly.
4. If you have the urge to cry, let the tears flow.
5. If you need to talk, find a good listener.
6. If grief is distracting you from your caregiving duties, see a professional counselor.

Helplessness: Helplessness is a hallmark of brain injury. Much of what will happen in your patient's recovery is beyond your control. You can't wake your survivor from her coma. You can't heal her brain. You can't accelerate her recovery; it is a slow, lifelong process. Worst of all, you can't foresee the future. No one knows how well your patient will recover.

Helplessness can be maddening. More importantly, it can lead to lethargy.

This situation is so bad.

There's nothing I can do to help.

I guess I'll stop trying.

Here are five ways to combat helplessness:

1. Identify what you can control. The Checklists for Success on pages 68, 105, 146, 178, and 209 are a great place to start.
2. Record your goals.
3. Plan how you will accomplish these goals.
4. Concentrate your energy on implementing these plans.
5. When helplessness resurfaces, refer to your list, your goals, and your plans, and put yourself back on track.

Loneliness: Only those who have experienced brain injury can truly appreciate the unique challenges you face. Your relatives and friends won't fully understand what you're going through. They may not know how to support you.

When loneliness is weakening your resolve, try these five suggestions:

1. Reach out to others. Ask for their support.
2. Explain that your survivor has been transformed forever and you have no idea what the future will bring.

3. Ask those closest to you to read this book.
4. Join a support group, either locally or online.
5. Don't go through this ordeal alone.

Fear: Fear is another potentially debilitating emotion. Brain injury can cause a multitude of fears, for example:

- Your patient may not recover as well as you hope.
- You may lose your job if you spend too much time at the hospital.
- The medical bills may bankrupt you.
- Your family may fall apart.
- You may not be up to the role of caregiver.
- You are terrified by the unknown.

Unresolved fears will eat away at you and compromise your ability to care for your survivor. Fear is best countered with education and action. If the unknown is keeping you awake at night, follow these eight suggestions:

1. Identify and confront your fears.
2. Absorb the information contained in this book.
3. Review and follow the advice offered.
4. If you need to know more, consult the List of Essential Resources on page 229.
5. If you're worried about money, read "Paying the Bills" on page 115. Then, review your finances and adjust your spending, if possible.
6. If your survivor is eligible for government benefits, apply now.
7. Be sure your employer fully grasps what you're going through.
8. If you're worried about your caregiving abilities, honestly assess your shortcomings and start asking for help. (See page 92.)

Depression: Unless you always view the glass as half-full, expect to be hit by depression soon, if it hasn't hit already. This is natural. The loss you suffered is shattering. The task ahead appears insurmountable.

Some depression is okay, but don't let your brain become habituated to depression. The actual mix of chemicals produced by your body when you are depressed can be tough to turn off if it flows for too long.

If depression is making it difficult for you to get out of bed in the morning, driving you to drink too much, or interfering with your caregiving, follow these four suggestions:

1. View your depression as the first step in adjusting to your loved one's brain injury.
2. Share your concerns and grief with somebody.
3. Seek professional counseling.
4. Tell your doctor about your depression and its causes. The temporary use of prescription medication can help lift the cloud of despair and re-energize you.

A major turning point for every caregiver is being able to conquer much of the anger, guilt, grief, helplessness, loneliness, fear, and depression that accompany this major, unanticipated life change. (These emotions will never go away completely.)

To be an excellent caregiver, you must trade your negative emotions for feelings that will focus your energy on supporting and advocating for your survivor. These are:

Joy   **Hope**   **Determination**

Joy: I know it's not easy to imagine feeling joy in the face of the daunting challenges you and your loved one face. However, it's crucial that your patient—who may sense and mimic your state of mind—be surrounded by positive energy.

Even today, Jessica is quick to recognize my moments of emotional turmoil and adopt my mood. Don't let your negative thinking thwart your survivor's progress. Keep these four suggestions in mind:

1. Celebrate even the tiniest gains—the first opening of an eye, the first spoken word, the first hug, the first meal.
2. Don't dwell on what your survivor was able to do before her injury.
3. Focus on what she can do now and the huge advances she will make in rehabilitation.
4. Remind yourself frequently that countless survivors of serious brain injuries create new, rewarding, and happy lives after their recovery and rehabilitation.

Hope: Hope is essential to a successful recovery. Without hope there is helplessness. When you're dragged down by helplessness, the rigors of living with a brain injury soon will exhaust you. Without hope, you become one more obstacle for your survivor. With hope, you can motivate her to work hard at her recovery and rehabilitation.

Some overly cautious doctors and nurses will try to stifle your hope by mistaking your realistic optimism for denial. Don't let them. But remember, there can be a fine line between hope and denial. A successful recovery is not a full recovery, but considerable headway is possible with perseverance and patience by the survivor and the unending support of her family and friends.

Determination: Your loved one is facing a monumental task. Her success depends on her determination to work hard and your determination to support her in every way possible.

To summarize the main points of this section, there are eight different ways you should be preparing yourself to be the caregiver your survivor deserves:

1. Focus on what you can control.
2. Take excellent care of yourself, both physically and emotionally.
3. Learn all you can about your survivor's brain injury.
4. Take regular vacations from your caregiving duties, even if just for a day.
5. Ask for help often.
6. Turn unhealthy emotions into an optimistic outlook.
7. Focus on the strength and resilience you share with your survivor.
8. Always remember, you can do this.

Faith

For many caregivers, the comfort and strength they derive from their faith gives them the joy, hope, and determination they need to excel at their new responsibilities.

For certain believers, however, a brain injury is a formidable challenge to their faith. "Why me?" they ask. "What did I do to deserve this misfortune?" They struggle to make sense of their lives, suddenly filled with disheartening and undeserved new trials. These feelings of abandonment can undermine their value as a caregiver.

If your survivor's brain injury has you doubting your faith, consider the following twelve suggestions:

1. Be open to the renewal of your faith.
2. Think back to a time when you felt the loving presence of God.
3. Pray, even if you doubt its usefulness.

4. Ask others to pray for you.
5. Attend services.
6. Try to identify and confront the emotions that may be overpowering your faith.
7. Remember, it's okay to be angry with God.
8. Talk to someone of faith whom you respect and trust; speak honestly about what has stolen your faith.
9. Talk to others who faced challenges and kept or regained their faith.
10. Stop asking "Why me?" There is no answer to this question.
11. Be mindful of the blessings you have been given.
12. Surround yourself with spiritual experiences: uplifting and inspirational music, books, poetry, and talks.

Asking for Help

Supporting a person with a brain injury through her grueling recovery and rehabilitation is more than a full-time job. Most of us can't devote all our time and energy to our survivor. We have responsibilities to our children, to our employers, or both. In my case, poor health forced me to be a part-time helper.

Even if you have no other responsibilities and are available full-time to support your survivor, spending every hour of every day at the hospital is a poor decision for nearly everyone. This is exhausting work. Fatigue inevitably leads to illness, and an ailing caregiver is a poor caregiver.

Recognize that you need help.

People will be willing, even eager, to help you and your survivor. They may even feel honored that you turned to them in a crisis. Give these folks the opportunity to help. Accept their assistance without embarrassment. Someday, you will be able to return the favor or aid someone else in need.

I asked everyone we knew for help and I was gratified by the response. A few "close" friends disappeared, and it hurt. But, you should expect this.

To make your requests for help easier and more productive, here are nine suggestions:

1. **Identify and record your needs.** My biggest need was for people to spend the afternoon with Jessica at the rehab facility. They encouraged her in her therapy, reminded her to rest between sessions, and cheered her when she became discouraged. You may need folks to

   - Compile information on brain injury.
   - Review your insurance policies.
   - Help you select a rehab facility.
   - Sit with your survivor.
   - Provide transportation.
   - Prepare meals.
   - Baby-sit or check on folks and animals at home.
   - Run errands.
   - Clean the house.
   - Mow the lawn.
   - Shovel the driveway.
   - What else do you need?

2. **Broadcast your needs widely.** People lead busy lives. They won't always be available when you need them. Here are five easy ways to reach everyone:

   - Send emails.
   - Record a message on your answering machine or voicemail.
   - Form a telephone tree.
   - Ask someone to organize a network of helpers and schedule their activities for you.

- Create a Web site to post the latest news. You can do this for free at www.CaringBridge.org and www.CarePages.com.

3. **Be prepared with a list of needs.** When people ask, "What can I do to help?" pull out your list and put them to work. People will stop asking if their initial offers are not accepted.

4. **Give people permission to say no.** In an email, I wrote, "I plan to ask for your support soon. This is difficult for me. You can make it easier by simply and directly saying 'No' when you're not available, for any reason. I promise I won't be hurt and I'll keep asking."

5. **Find the right man or woman for the job.** Jessica's well-read Uncle Elliot was unable to spend a full afternoon at the rehab hospital. He was, however, the ideal person to find me a few books about brain injury rehabilitation.

6. **Be creative.** There are all kinds of ways people can help. Jessica's cousin, Lisa, was housebound with a complicated pregnancy. From her bed, she maintained the ever-growing list of folks receiving my emails. Lisa circulated the messages and compiled the responses. This saved me hours of aggravation.

7. **Let others perform tasks that may upset you.** On the day of Jessica's accident, the hospital social worker handed me a plastic bag containing Jessica's clothing. I discarded the bag because I couldn't bear to open it. Six months later, we realized that the bag I discarded probably contained a cherished necklace. It didn't occur to me at the time to set the bag aside and ask someone to check its contents.

8. **Keep asking for help as long as you need it, even if others question you.** About six weeks after Jessica's accident, my mother asked, "Don't these people have families of their own to care for?" I think she was embarrassed by my frequent appeals for help. I learned, however, that many people were happy to support and to continue supporting Jessica's recovery.

9. **Periodically ask someone if you have overlooked something that will help your survivor.** In my discombobulation, I didn't think to bring Jessica her favorite foods when she was in rehabilitation. I also learned too late—from Karen Brennan's moving memoir, *Being with Rachel: A Story of Memory and Survival*—how much Jessica might have benefited from my cuddling in bed with her. What are you overlooking?

The Family and Medical Leave Act

The Family and Medical Leave Act may allow you to spend more time with your patient without jeopardizing your job. This law permits certain employees to take unpaid, job-protected leave from work to care for an immediate family member (spouse, child, or parent) who has a serious health condition.

Here's what you need to know about the Family and Medical Leave Act:

- You are covered by this legislation if you meet all five of these conditions:

  1. Your employer has fifty or more employees working within seventy-five miles of your job site.
  2. You have been on the job for at least one year.

3. You have worked for your employer for at least 1,250 hours in the preceding year.
4. You have exhausted your sick and vacation leave.
5. You intend to return to your job following this permitted absence.

- You may use this leave time to:

    o Help your survivor with basic medical, hygiene, safety, and nutritional needs.
    o Accompany her to appointments with physicians and other health care professionals.
    o Support her in her occupational, physical, and speech therapy sessions.
    o Arrange for changes in care, such as transferring her from the hospital to a rehabilitation facility.

- The law allows you to use twelve weeks of family and medical leave each year, taken either all at once or at intervals throughout the year.

- Employers are not obligated to pay your wages when you are caring for your loved one. This, unfortunately, prevents many caregivers from benefiting from this law.

- Your employer must continue to provide the same benefits—including your health insurance—when you miss work to care for an ailing family member.

- The law stipulates that you request leave at least thirty days in advance, though it allows notice to be given as soon as practicable when unforeseen events, such as a brain injury, arise.

- A 2008 extension to this Act permits a spouse, son, daughter, parent, or next of kin to take up to twenty-six weeks of unpaid, job-protected leave to care for a member of the Armed Forces, including the National Guard and Reserves, who is undergoing medical treatment, recuperation, or therapy; is in outpatient status; or is otherwise on the temporary disability retired list, for a serious injury or illness.

- This extension also permits an employee to take twelve weeks of unpaid leave to address certain issues that may occur when a relative is called to active duty or notified of an impending call to active duty. These include, but are not limited to attending certain military events, arranging for childcare, making some financial and legal arrangements, attending certain counseling sessions, and receiving post-employment reintegration briefings.

- Some states have laws that provide rights in addition to those authorized by the federal law.

- Employers may try to ignore the Family and Medical Leave Act. If this happens to you, you have the right to enact legal proceedings.

- Employers have been known to retaliate against workers who use this leave. Beware if this sounds like your boss.

- You can read more about the Family and Medical Leave Act at www.dol.gov/esa/whd/fmla.

- To locate the U.S. Department of Labor office in your area that will answer your questions about the FMLA call 866-487-9243.

Case Managers

A brain injury case manager is a health care professional—usually a nurse, a rehab counselor, or a social worker—whose job is to manage health care services and advocate for their clients and their families. The goals of a case manager are to help their clients:

- Maximize the use of available benefits, resources, and services.
- Recover to the best of their ability.
- Live as independently as possible.
- Smoothly integrate back into the community.
- Enjoy the highest quality of life.
- Achieve these goals in a cost-effective way.

In short, you and a case manager share the same goals for your loved one. A good case manager, however, has the time, knowledge, skills, and experience to accomplish these goals.

Ideally, case management should start within weeks of the injury. But, it can begin and end at any time throughout the lifelong recovery process.

A case manager provides a wide range of services tailored to the requirements of the survivor and her family. Here are some things a case manager can do for you and your survivor:

- Assess your loved one's condition and needs in the following areas: medical, rehabilitation, insurance, legal, recreational, vocational, educational, housing, social, psychological, and behavioral.
- Develop and coordinate an integrated plan to address these needs.
- Consider both the short-term and the long-term.

- Locate health care providers and services, such as rehab facilities, physicians, therapists, and counselors.
- Research and recommend support groups, attorneys, respite care, and alternative living arrangements.
- Identify relevant government and community programs, benefits, and services, such as disability income, vocational training, and special education.
- Contract, monitor, and evaluate services.
- Interact with physicians, therapists, attorneys, insurance adjusters, employers, teachers, and others.
- Manage the transfer of the patient from one facility to another, such as from the ICU to the general ward of the hospital or from the hospital to a rehab facility.
- Prepare the family for the patient's homecoming and recommend any home modifications to accommodate the survivor's special needs.
- Educate the family about brain injury.
- Act as an expert witness in court cases.

How Do I Find a Case Manager?

When your survivor is in the hospital, at an inpatient rehabilitation facility, or participating in a day rehab program, there will be an in-house social worker or case manager who will negotiate with your health insurer, and, perhaps, perform a few of the other services listed above. This varies widely among facilities.

Your health insurance company may provide a case manager to oversee reimbursable medical services. His loyalty, however, lies with his employer, not you and your survivor. He, almost certainly, will be stingy with his company's money.

Some state brain injury associations (see page 234) provide case management services. This should be the first place you call. If they don't provide the services your survivor requires, they may be able to recommend someone who does. Some state and local governments offer case management services. Check the blue pages in your phone book.

With more people surviving brain injuries, a new industry of brain injury case management services has emerged. These professionals usually charge an hourly fee for their services, plus expenses. To locate one in your area, look in the yellow pages under "Rehabilitation Services."

Here are some things to consider when hiring a case manager:

Credentials

- Is she licensed in her profession?
- Is she certified by the Academy of Certified Brain Injury Specialists?

Experience

- How long has she represented brain injury survivors?
- How many individuals and families has she helped?
- Will she provide references?
- Does she sound well informed about brain injury?
- Does she understand the issues you're facing?

Costs

- What is her fee and expenses?
- What does she estimate your total charges will be?
- Does she offer a sliding scale based on income?

Compatibility

- Will you and your survivor feel comfortable working with her for weeks, months, and, possibly, years?

Availability

- When is she available for consultations?
- How frequently will she communicate with you?
- Will she communicate with you in person, telephone, email, and/or fax?

How Well Will My Survivor Recover?

One of the unsettling realities of brain injury is the uncertainty. No one knows how well your survivor will recover. The brain is a complex, wondrous organ that remains much of a mystery to doctors and scientists. Many variables—biological, chemical, physiological, genetic, psychological, cultural, social, academic, financial, familial, vocational, and community—impact how well someone recovers from a brain injury. This uncertainty places a heavy burden on physicians who face families desperate for a glimpse of the future.

Some doctors offer a pessimistic perspective. Their reasoning: the family should prepare for the worst and be pleased with anything that exceeds a catastrophic outcome. They also may fear a lawsuit if the patient fails to meet expectations. Plenty of survivors surpass these bleak prognoses, and their families are pleased. But this strategy can crush the hope a caregiver needs to inspire and encourage her survivor to achieve the best possible outcome.

For just this reason, other doctors offer a more optimistic picture. Their aim is to support the family through the trying months ahead. As one mother on the panel told me, "False hope is better than no hope."

This strategy also has its downside. A second mother, after being assured her son would be able to return to college, was devastated when his persistent cognitive impairments burst her unrealistic view of his academic future.

I just as easily could have been distraught, if I took to heart the well-intended comment by Dr. Thomas that Jessica may be able to resume her career.

A third group of doctors stick to the Litany of Uncertainty (see page 49) and refuse to offer any prognosis. This works for certain families. They prefer to live day to day, concentrating on the care and comfort of their survivor. One father told me, "In my case, ignorance was bliss. I didn't want to know how bad it might be. Nor, did I want to develop any false hopes."

While some folks do okay not knowing, many of us can't help but imagine the future. We yearn for something realistic—and a bit optimistic—to cling to. We research the possibilities and the probabilities, the worst case and the best case, expecting our survivor's outcome to fall somewhere in between.

While it's impossible to predict the future for any single patient, the science of brain injury has advanced so that doctors now can discuss probable outcomes with some confidence. Researchers have identified the factors that influence the success of a patient's recovery. Reviewing these factors with your doctor can provide at least a hazy picture of the future.

Bearing in mind that every brain injury is unique and unpredictable, you may want to reflect on the following list.

Factors that Impact the Success of Recovery from a Brain Injury

- The nature, location, and gravity of the injury
- How soon the injury is diagnosed
- The quality and speed of acute care
- The depth and duration of the coma
- The length of post-traumatic amnesia
- How rapidly the patient proceeds through the stages of the Glasgow Coma Scale and the Rancho Los Amigos Scale of Cognitive Functioning
- The patient's age

- How quickly the patient begins rehabilitation
- The quality and quantity of rehabilitative care
- The nature and extent of other injuries
- The quality and quantity of the involvement of family and friends
- The extent to which the patient and caregiver use easily available resources, such as support groups, educational materials, and community programs
- The patient's pre-injury physical and mental health
- The degree of the patient's education
- The individual's past history of alcohol and/or substance abuse
- The ability of the survivor and her caregiver to recognize and adapt to the reality that the individual will not return to her pre-injury condition
- The spiritual comfort of the survivor and her caregiver
- The individual's personality, including her

  o Ability to cope with adversity
  o Self-control and patience
  o Flexibility
  o Determination
  o Intelligence and intellectual curiosity
  o Motivation to succeed
  o Engagement in life

The maxim, "Use it or lose it" applies well to brain injury. A survivor who has lived an active, challenging, and full pre-injury life has conditioned her brain to be well-prepared for the rigorous reworking necessary to recover well. A patient who perseveres in her rehabilitation, in the challenges of daily life, and in the pursuit of an active and productive lifestyle will give her brain the exercise it needs to heal.

Notes

Checklist for Success #2
Focus on What You Can Control

___ Have you found an easy way to keep family and friends up to date on your survivor's condition? [See page 93.]

___ Caregiving is a grueling job. Have you begun to take care of yourself?

- Eat healthful regular meals.
- Exercise.
- Get enough sleep.
- Harness your emotions. [See page 83.]
- Do what sustains you, such as listening to music or walking in the woods, to recover some of the energy you have been expending.
- Ask for help from family and friends. [See page 92.]
- Join a support group either online or locally. [See page 231.]

___ Are you learning about your survivor's brain injury? If reading this book is not enough, check out the List of Essential Resources on page 229.

___ Are you aware that the Family and Medical Leave Act may allow you to spend more time with your survivor without jeopardizing your job? For the details, see page 95.

___ Is your faith supporting or undermining your efforts to be an excellent caregiver? If you're feeling abandoned by your faith, see page 91.

____ Have you begun to advocate for your survivor?

- Make yourself an equal member of your survivor's medical team.
- Learn the ropes; how does your hospital and medical team operate?
- Learn the jargon; consult the Glossary on page 219.
- Don't be afraid to ask questions.
- Are you receiving a clear explanation of your survivor's condition and a realistic picture of the future?
- Is your survivor receiving the best care possible? Speak up if you are unhappy with this care.
- If the hospital has a patient advocate, contact this person if you have concerns about your survivor's treatment.

____ Have you considered hiring a brain injury case manager to help you care for your survivor? [See page 98.]

____ Have you begun to compile a list of possible rehabilitation facilities for your survivor? [See page 196]

____ Do you know what factors impact a successful recovery from a brain injury? If not, see page 102. Have you reviewed this list to see which items you can control?

____ Have you begun to adjust to the fact that a successful recovery from a serious brain injury is not a full recovery?

9

Waiting, Watching, Hoping
Emerging from a Coma

The sixth day of our around-the-clock vigil of waiting, watching, and hoping started much like the previous days. Family and friends were still camped out in the hospital, in nearby hotels, and in our home. Jessica still was in a coma.

With folks congregating in our tiny room outside the ICU, my sister Barbara and I rested at home for a few hours after lunch. For the first time since the accident, I was able to nap during the day.

When Barbara and I arrived back at the hospital we were shocked to find a new family in our private waiting room. Our distress turned to quiet panic when we couldn't find any familiar faces. Barbara and I grudgingly moved into the much larger, much less private ICU waiting room. We sat down in a state of turmoil, though Barbara hid her feelings well.

Our private room was occupied by others. The twenty-four hour vigil at Jessica's bedside apparently was over. In my frazzled state, I couldn't help but conclude that Jessica had died while I rested.

For two or three minutes, Barbara and I sat paralyzed with fear before thinking to ask a nurse about Jessica's condition, which, thankfully—at least this time—was unchanged.

Thirty minutes later, Jessica's family poured into the waiting room, oblivious to our alarm. Robert explained that a new patient had been brought into the ICU and his family now would have the privacy we had for nearly a week.

Also, a nurse had told Robert that Jessica was having another series of CT scans and would be unavailable to visitors for two hours. For the first time, Jessica's family was able to enjoy a meal together. It just hadn't occurred to anyone to stay nearby to insulate me from the shock of finding our private room occupied by others.

This omission is not surprising. When Jessica's family gets together, she usually directs the action, at least as well as this unruly clan accepts direction. With Jessica in a coma, there was no heir apparent to take control. As Jessica's youngest sister Kathy wondered, "Who's going to keep this family together? Who's going to be our mom?"

That evening, I realized that once Jessica's condition had stabilized, three days after her injury, I should have urged her brothers and sisters to head home. They could have saved precious hours of leave from work to visit another time when Jessica and I needed their support much more. This is yet another of the lessons I learned too late.

When I entered the spacious, dark, and dreary ICU waiting room, I noticed its occupants had separated themselves into seven groups. Each cluster comprised the family and friends of a patient in the unit. We moved into the sole vacant space, bringing with us any of the unclaimed, well-worn furniture. Jessica's oldest brother Joe dragged over a creaky, faded recliner for me to stretch out and ease my aching muscles.

A telephone was located near a wall of large windows facing a bank of heating and air-conditioning units. Whoever answered the constantly ringing phone called out a patient's name. A member of that family crossed the room to take the call. Watching this procession, we soon learned the names of the seven other families. In the same manner, they soon recognized us as the "Jessica family."

An hour after we had settled into our new home, we were approached by a waiting-room neighbor. After introducing herself and telling me about her husband's stroke, she asked about Jessica's condition and prognosis. Soon, information about Jessica's brain injury passed from group to group.

In the early afternoon of the next day, as I was returning to my recliner after a brief visit with Jessica, I was intercepted by Ted. He pointed out his teenage daughter and son and shared with me the story of his wife's brain injury. Janet had been struck in the head by a passing car as she instinctively leaned into the road to retrieve a dropped package. Ted, a farmer, and his two teenagers were camped out in the waiting room. They had not been home—a five-hour drive south—since arriving a week earlier when Janet had been transferred from a hospital closer to home.

The next morning, I met Susan, whose husband Jim, a realtor, acquired his brain injury when his Lexus hydroplaned off the road. Susan, Ted, and I formed a spontaneous support group, three very different people with very different lives sharing the same fears. A brain injury is an instant equalizer in our heterogeneous society.

As Jessica's first week in the ICU ended, Dr. Thomas expressed disappointment that she still was not responding to commands.

Due to her intense pain, Jessica had been heavily sedated, which could extend her coma. Now, the nurses were reducing her pain medications and sedatives, and Jessica was becoming much more active.

Jessica could not remain in the hospital indefinitely. Within the next week or so, a decision had to be made regarding the next step in her treatment. If she emerged from her coma, Jessica would be transferred to a rehab facility. Otherwise, she would be parked in a nursing home. To be prepared, Barbara and I began to investigate the local nursing homes. We also began to worry about the quality of care Jessica would receive there.

With the prospect of a prolonged coma, paying the expenses of Jessica's care also became a concern. If she was transferred to a nursing home, our health insurance would not cover the costs.

On Jessica's ninth day in the ICU, Dr. Thomas prepared her for an extended coma. Since she had no spinal cord injury, he removed her cervical collar. He performed a *tracheotomy*, a minor surgical procedure in which an opening is cut in the neck, allowing the tube from the ventilator to be placed directly into the windpipe, rather than through the patient's mouth. He also inserted a feeding tube (a Gastric or G Tube) through Jessica's abdomen and directly into her stomach, allowing the tube threaded through her nose to be removed.

Physical therapists splinted Jessica's arms, legs, and feet to prevent her from clenching them and to reduce *spasticity*, which is the excessive, and potentially permanent, tightening of muscles, tendons, and ligaments. Spasticity can result in long-term harm, limited mobility, and pain. The physical therapists also taught us to move Jessica's arms and legs through range-of-motion exercises to guard against extensive muscle loss.

While there was no change in Jessica's condition, she looked much better without the cumbersome cervical collar, the ventilator tube in her mouth, and the feeding tube passing through her nose. I had mixed feelings about this. On the upside, Jessica appeared to demand less machinery to keep her alive. On the downside, she looked like a person in a persistent vegetative state.

Dr. Zimmerman warned us that the extensive tearing of Jessica's brainstem could leave her in a coma for months. When I grumbled that our health insurance wouldn't cover the cost of custodial care, Dr. Zimmerman explained that comatose patients can receive reimbursable medical treatment if the doctors document active continuing therapy resulting in progress. He tried to encourage us with the story of a patient who was in a coma for three years and "woke up just fine."

The possibility of a prolonged coma elicited an even more crucial issue. Throughout our twenty years together, Jessica had made it clear she didn't want to be kept alive, indefinitely, by a machine. I recognized that if this situation arose, I might not be willing to let her go. I asked my sister Barbara and our friend Michael to argue Jessica's case if it became clear that her brainstem would not heal; the burdens we sometimes place on family and friends.

Dr. Thomas remained guarded whenever we asked about Jessica's long-term prognosis. He was a taciturn physician from the old school. He was treating Jessica as best he could. We had great faith in his medical skills, but he saw little cause to involve us in the complexities of the case. He prohibited our family physician from reviewing Jessica's medical chart— *Strike 1.* He was insistent we not speculate about Jessica's long-term outcome, as if that was even remotely possible—*Strike 2.* When we began to ask questions, revealing our attempts to educate ourselves, Dr. Thomas responded with abrupt, condescending answers—*Strike 3.*

Gaining no information from the Chief of Trauma Services, we grabbed every opportunity to talk to the other doctors treating Jessica. Like Dr. Thomas, they usually recited from the Litany of Uncertainty or gave vague and inconclusive responses. Occasionally, when pressed, they were more forthcoming, though they always qualified their responses as merely "best guesses."

Brain injuries are complex. In a way, this is a new field of medicine as people now survive traumas that a decade or two earlier would have killed them. Dr. Thomas truly was unable to answer our questions with anything but his best guess. As head honcho, he must have felt that his words must be far more definitive than a best guess.

Unfortunately, there was nothing Jessica's doctors could do to wake her. We simply had to wait for her brainstem to heal.

For the first time in my relationship with Jessica, I was powerless to influence her well-being. I had unwillingly yielded that capacity to God and Dr. Thomas, and my relationships with both needed work. My fears, frustrations, and anger, which I felt intensely at the time and still tearfully recollect today, demanded an outlet. Dr. Thomas provided an easy target.

If only he was more forthcoming, I thought, *this ordeal would be more bearable.*

But then he surprised me.

Ten days after her accident, without warning, Jessica was transferred from the ICU to the Intermediate Care Unit (IMC). Was this a sign of progress in her condition? Or, was this transfer due to the pending arrival of a new patient who had a greater need for Jessica's ICU bed? I wasn't told. When I returned to the ICU after dinner, I was stunned to find her room vacant.

Much of my concern with the transfer was the buzz in the ICU waiting room that the level of care drops considerably when a patient is moved to the IMC. It was rumored—groundlessly, but credibly to me in my hypersensitive state—that the family was expected to provide some care for the patient. With my disabilities, I was afraid I wouldn't be able to care for Jessica. This misimpression was reinforced when I noticed that the IMC nurses had not been notified that Jessica was to receive limited stimulation.

Apparently, my discomfort was reported to Dr. Thomas. He found me, still shaken, in a corner of the IMC waiting room. He assured me that Jessica would be well cared for by the nurses. If I had any concerns, he said, I should call him immediately.

The next morning during rounds, Dr. Thomas greeted me warmly. As he discussed Jessica's case, he shocked the nurses by instructing them to "be sure to wash her hair today." He then asked me if I had any issues to discuss. I later learned that Dr. Thomas rarely mentioned the personal care of a patient or invited input from a spouse during rounds.

Of the three patients in the unit with brain injuries, only Jessica and Susan's husband, Jim, moved on to the next step in their recovery. When it became clear that Janet wouldn't recover from her blow to the head, our bond with Ted was broken and our informal support group dissolved. We no longer shared the same emotions. Susan and I still had hope. Ted would soon be planning a funeral. Just the sight of us added to Ted's grief, and we were at a loss for words to console him.

Notes

10

Paying the Bills
Health Insurance, Disability Pay, and Attorneys

If you haven't already begun thinking about your household finances, now is the time. You need to minimize the amount of money going out for medical expenses and maximize the amount coming in through disability pay. To accomplish this, you may want to hire an attorney. This chapter helps you sort through these issues.

Health Insurance

When it comes to treating survivors of a brain injury, our health care system is unkind and shortsighted. The medical costs of recovery and rehabilitation can be astronomical. A patient with a severe brain injury and her health insurer easily can spend millions for her care. Acting early to understand the costs you are facing and the insurance benefits available to your survivor may help you avoid financial distress.

Health insurance—if you have it—generally covers much, if not most, of a survivor's medical care during the acute stage of recovery. Then, it gets tricky. To recover well, every survivor of a serious brain injury must undergo extensive rehabilitation. This includes the standard physical, speech, occupational, and neuropsychological therapy, plus the newer cognitive rehabilitation.

In *Confronting Traumatic Brain Injury: Devastation, Hope, and Healing*—a forceful indictment of government, insurance, and medical policy regarding brain injury—William J. Winslade writes that most survivors do not receive adequate rehabilitation. This is shortsighted, he argues, since "a relatively few dollars spent on rehabilitation could make the difference between a life of dependency and one of relatively full function."

With their eyes on the bottom line, health insurers limit what they pay for rehabilitation, both inpatient and outpatient. They typically pay for just two to six weeks of inpatient rehabilitation. Even worse, they sometimes insist that inpatient rehab be completed within a certain period of time, within ninety days of the injury, for example. This can be a big problem if your patient is slow to emerge from her coma.

With outpatient rehabilitation, health insurers usually cap the number of reimbursable physical, speech, and occupational therapy sessions at twenty-five to fifty per year or, even worse, per injury. With cognitive rehabilitation, they are even stingier.

The impairments most disabling to most survivors of a brain injury are deficits in attention, concentration, memory, problem-solving, and decision-making. Cognitive rehabilitation is the best way to remediate these complaints. Insurance companies, however, often deny payment, claiming that there is no evidence that cognitive rehabilitation is effective. Recent research, however, has concluded otherwise and the Brain Injury Association of America is leading the fight to have cognitive rehabilitation recognized by the insurance industry as standard, reimbursable treatment for a brain injury.

Many health insurance policies also have lifetime benefit caps, such as $1,000,000, that are easily exceeded with a serious brain injury. Caregivers often find that just when their survivor is benefiting the most from rehabilitation, the insurance company says, "No more."

Every rehab program has a case manager who negotiates with the health insurer over the amount of reimbursable services. Your survivor is best served if the case manager at the rehabilitation facility you select has many years of successful experience working with health insurers.

If you fear that your health insurance benefits may be lacking, consider these nine ways to maximize them:

1. If you have not already informed your survivor's health insurer about her injury, do it now.

2. If you have not been assigned a case manager at the hospital or rehab facility, ask for one.

3. Cultivate a good working relationship with this person.

4. Review your policy carefully, or

5. Have an insurance expert, an independent case manager, or an attorney who specializes in personal injury litigation review your policy.

6. Ask about extra-contractual or going-out-of-contract exceptions that may be mutually beneficial to insurer and patient. For example, all parties involved may agree that it's best to cut short inpatient rehab provided the insurer picks up the tab for seventy-five, rather than fifty, annual outpatient rehab sessions. Be sure to get any extra-contractual agreements in writing.

7. Be sure your doctors are documenting all progress in your family member's condition, even the tiniest. Health insurers are quick to stop payment if the patient is not progressing.

8. If you feel your insurer is not treating you fairly, file an appeal with the company.

9. If your appeal is denied, speak to an attorney.

When your health insurer says, "No more," check out these potential sources of financial assistance for your medical bills:

- Medicaid, if your income and financial assets are small (See page 120.)

- Hospital patient assistance programs for people with low incomes: Talk to the hospital billing department. They may work with you to establish a payment plan you can afford.

- Medicare, if your survivor qualifies for Social Security Disability Income: Medicare benefits, however, don't begin until two years after the injury. (See page 121.)

- Auto insurance, if the injury was the result of a car accident

- Workers' Compensation, if the injury occurred at work (See page 132.)

- Homeowners insurance, if the injury occurred at your house or someone else's

- If it's possible someone other than your survivor was responsible for the injury, see an attorney.

- State programs, such as:

  o Brain injury trust funds
  o Occupational and vocational rehabilitation services
  o Crime victim's compensation
  o Medical assistance
  o Developmental disabilities for children
  o A high risk insurance pool for uninsurable people
  o Note that every state is different. For information about programs in your state, contact your state brain injury association (see page 234).

- Tell your doctors you're having financial problems. They may give you a break on their fees.

- Surf the Web for federal, state, and local government assistance programs. Try www.GovBenefits.gov.

- Apply for assistance from charitable and civic organizations.

- Follow the example of many brain injury families who have had raffles, yard sales, car washes, bake sales, road races, and concerts to raise funds for their survivor's medical expenses.

- Finally, don't forget that your medical expenses may be tax deductible.

Medicaid

Medicaid is a joint federal and state health insurance program that assists low-income people who do not have health insurance or who have exhausted their benefits. You are eligible for Medicaid if you meet certain financial requirements. Here's what you need to know:

- Medicaid rules are complex and they change frequently.

- Each state, within broad national guidelines, establishes its own eligibility criteria: the type, duration, amount, and scope of the medical services reimbursed; and the individual's co-payments.

- The eligibility requirements for Medicaid include the survivor's age, the amount of her income and financial assets, and whether she is a citizen or a lawfully admitted immigrant.

- The applicant must have few financial assets. A married couple may have approximately $2,000 to $5,000 in savings. Their home and one vehicle are exempt.

- To apply for Medicaid, contact your local or state government Medicaid office. See the blue pages of your telephone directory.

- Apply as soon as possible; approval takes a long time.

- For help with your application, you may want to hire an attorney, a case manager, or other professional with Medicaid expertise.

- Some states have additional "state-only" programs that provide medical assistance for certain low income people who don't qualify for Medicaid.

- Since most states must balance their books, Medicaid services—the second largest item in the budget after schools—are regularly reduced or eliminated altogether.

- For years, people with too many financial assets to qualify for Medicaid transferred some or all of their assets to relatives before applying. There now is a five-year "look-back" period that guards against these fraudulent transfers.

Some states have waivers that authorize them to provide, through Medicaid, an array of services, such as personal care attendants, home health care, case management, and respite care. These waivers are designed to enable individuals to live at home or in a community-based setting, rather than in a more costly institution.

Certain states even include cognitive rehabilitation on the menu of services offered with a Medicaid waiver. Beware that the eligibility criteria for a Medicaid waiver sometime defy logic. For example, in some states the survivor must have been injured after the age of sixteen.

Medicare

Medicare is the nation's largest health insurance program. The majority of Medicare recipients are sixty-five years of age or older. Also eligible for Medicare are people who have received Social Security Disability Income (see page 125) for two years. While twenty-four months may seem to be a long way off, you should be familiar with this program for your long-term

121

financial planning. Here's what you need to know about Medicare:

- Medicare has three parts:

    1. **Part A** - Hospital Insurance covers inpatient care in hospitals and skilled nursing facilities and some home health care. Most recipients don't pay for Part A because they or a spouse paid Medicare taxes while they were working.

    2. **Part B** - Medical Insurance covers doctors' services, outpatient care, and other medical services not covered by Part A, such as physical, occupational, and speech therapy. Nearly all recipients pay a standard monthly premium ($96.40 in 2009) for Part B. This premium usually is deducted from your monthly Social Security Disability Income benefit.

    3. **Part D** - The Medicare Prescription Drug Plan is optional. If you do not purchase Part D when you initially qualify for Medicare and decide to buy it later, you may pay a penalty. The cost varies depending on which provider you select. You may be able to choose a plan with no monthly premium.

- You choose how to have your medical services covered by Medicare. You can select either the original Medicare plan or you can choose among a number of Health Maintenance Organizations (HMOs) or Preferred Provider Organizations (PPOs) that participate in the Medicare Advantage program. Selecting among the Medicare Advantage plans is a time-consuming, complex exercise, but it can save you some money.

- Each year, you can review your health and prescription needs and switch to an alternative Medicare plan in the fall.

- If you have limited income and financial assets, your state may pay some or all of your Medicare premiums, deductibles, and coinsurance.

- You can learn more about Medicare by calling 800-633-4227 or visiting www.medicare.gov.

Disability Pay

With a serious brain injury, your survivor is certain to miss a long period of work, and possibly, never work again. Obviously, this can be a huge drain on the family budget. Now is the time to plan for this financial blow.

Most of us, lacking the foresight and/or finances to purchase a private disability insurance policy, are dependent on our employer, the federal government, and our coworkers, to offset a medical disability. Let's begin with your survivor's employer.

Disability Insurance at Work

You may be wondering how many more paychecks your patient will receive now that she's unable to work. The answer depends upon four circumstances:

1. How much sick and vacation time she has accumulated: Usually, this is a few days, weeks, or months.

2. Whether her employer provides short-term disability benefits: Short-term disability generally covers the first six months of absence.

3. Whether her employer provides long-term disability (LTD) benefits: LTD usually kicks in after six months of absence and continues until retirement age.

4. Whether her employer has a leave sharing program

Jessica was fortunate to have LTD benefits at work. She collects monthly disability checks that pay two-thirds of her salary—the industry standard—at the time of her injury. These checks started 180 days after her injury. Like most recipients, we pay taxes on these LTD benefits as earned income.

Long-term disability insurers typically deduct from the monthly benefit any other disability pay collected by the insured, such as Social Security Disability Income (SSDI) or Workers' Compensation.

If your survivor will receive LTD benefits, you may see no reason to apply for SSDI. You should for three reasons:

1. The LTD insurer probably will require it. If your survivor collects SSDI, the insurance company saves big bucks. They, likely, will even pay for an attorney to help your survivor obtain SSDI. If they don't offer, ask.

2. LTD plans—unlike SSDI—typically do not have cost-of-living adjustments. Jessica will collect the same monthly LTD benefit until she reaches retirement age. Each year, inflation nibbles away at the purchasing power of her benefit. The LTD provider generally will not deduct the annual Social Security cost-of-living adjustment from the benefit they pay your survivor. So, with SSDI, your individual's overall disability benefit will increase a bit most years.

3. Most importantly, individuals who receive SSDI are eligible for Medicare (see page 121), which will help you pay future medical bills.

Leave Sharing

Jessica's employer did not provide short-term disability insurance to cover the six-month gap between her injury and her LTD coverage. Fortunately, she had compassionate colleagues.

Many workplaces have leave sharing programs through which coworkers can contribute accrued leave—usually vacation, not sick pay—to colleagues who have medical emergencies, either themselves or within their families. Jessica's employer started a leave sharing program as a result of her accident. Thanks to the generosity of her colleagues, Jessica collected a full paycheck for months after her accident.

If I had still been working at the time of Jessica's injury, I would have qualified for my employer's leave sharing program as the spouse of an injured person.

If your survivor's employer does not have a leave sharing program, it can't hurt to ask her colleagues to start one, especially if she's well regarded.

Social Security Disability Income

A benefit available to everyone who has worked a certain number of years is Social Security Disability Income (SSDI). SSDI is not welfare. It is insurance you pay for your entire working life. Your loved one is entitled to these benefits.

Since the baby boomers are aging and the Social Security Administration (SSA) is woefully understaffed, filing for SSDI is a lengthy process. But, it's time well spent.

For me, filing for Jessica's SSDI was a welcome respite from the helplessness and anxiety I was experiencing at the time. I was able to lose myself in the details of the application and feel productive.

If you're too distracted to complete the application carefully—and it must be done carefully—ask someone to do it for you. Or, you can hire a case manager, an attorney, or other professional experienced in SSA procedures to apply for your survivor.

If you have not already done so, contact the Social Security Administration now (800-772-1213 & www.ssa.gov/disability) to begin the application process. If you prefer to speak to an SSA representative face to face, you can locate your local office in the blue pages of your phone book under United States Government.

Here's what you need to know about Social Security Disability Income:

- SSDI does not cover short-term or partial disability.

- To qualify, your survivor must have a medical condition that, in the opinion of the SSA, prevents her from working for at least a year.

- With most private disability insurance, the insured is entitled to benefits if she can no longer work at her current profession, for example, as an attorney or as a carpenter. SSDI requires that the applicant be unable to work at any job, or, in their words, at any "substantial gainful activity" which, in 2009, paid $980 per month.

- The SSA considers the following factors when determining whether one is able to work at substantial gainful activity: her medical condition, age, education, training, and daily activities before and after her injury.

- SSDI usually commences with the sixth month of disability and continues until retirement age.

- At retirement age, SSDI automatically converts to the standard Social Security benefit every worker is entitled to in her golden years. The amount of the monthly benefit does not change with this conversion.

- Given that months or years will pass before your survivor receives her first SSDI check, it will be a big one. Benefits are paid retroactive to the date of eligibility if the application is submitted within one year of the injury. Otherwise, benefits are paid retroactive to the date of application.

- The monthly SSDI benefit is based on the applicant's age and how much she has paid into the system. The average monthly benefit in 2009 was $1,153.

- About one-third of SSDI beneficiaries—those with higher incomes—pay income taxes on eighty-five percent of their benefit. People with lower incomes pay taxes on a smaller portion or pay no taxes at all.

- Each January, the SSDI benefit increases a small amount if the cost of living has risen.

- The amount of your financial assets has no impact on your eligibility. If Bill Gates acquired a serious brain injury, he would qualify for SSDI.

- The Social Security Administration determines if you are disabled, not your doctor. They require substantial medical proof of the disability and detailed descriptions of the claimant's capabilities and impairments.

- When you apply for disability benefits, the SSA may send you to a physician, at their expense, for a medical exam.

- Some spouses and/or children of SSDI beneficiaries are eligible for payments. The rules are complicated. Be sure to discuss your family situation with an SSA representative.

- Young men, the largest group of brain injury survivors, usually have not paid enough into the Social Security system to qualify for SSDI. They may, however, qualify for another program administered by the Social Security Administration, Supplemental Security Income, which is discussed on page 131.

- If your brain injury is labeled "mild," you must have extensive documentation of your impairments and much patience to qualify for Social Security Disability Income. In her humorous and insightful book, *I'll Carry the Fork! Recovering a Life after Brain Injury*, Kara Swanson describes her struggles to demonstrate her eligibility for SSDI with a mild brain injury.

- The majority of applicants for SSDI initially are rejected. If this happens to you, don't be discouraged; appeal the decision within sixty days.

Obtaining Social Security Disability Income is a long and frustrating, but ultimately fair, process. If your survivor is disabled by her brain injury, if she has the support of her health care providers, if you have completed the paperwork clearly and completely, and if you keep appealing, she should qualify for SSDI.

Appealing Your Case for SSDI

I applied for Jessica's SSDI one week after her car crash, when she was still in a coma. Four months later, when her application reached the top of the pile, the Social Security Administration denied her claim. They determined that:

- Jessica's condition was improving—*True*
- Jessica was alert and coherent—*Mostly true*
- Jessica was not expected to remain disabled for twelve consecutive months—*Certainly not true*

I filed for reconsideration on the grounds that Jessica's disability would last more than one year. Remember, you must file for reconsideration within sixty days of receiving your initial denial.

The initial application for SSDI by survivors of a brain injury usually is rejected for a combination of four reasons:

1. Brain injuries are complicated. Cognitive impairments, unlike physical deficits, are tough to detect and evaluate.

2. The SSA goal is to provide benefits quickly to the largest number of qualified applicants. They scan each application, approving only those that clearly meet the eligibility requirements. They deny applications that involve more time to evaluate.

3. Traumatic brain injury is not yet on the list of automatic disabling impairments used by the evaluators.

4. Doctor's offices and government bureaucracies often move slowly. All of the documentation required to prove the severity of a brain injury generally does not reach the evaluator prior to the initial ruling.

Successfully Surviving a Brain Injury

When a claimant requests reconsideration, the SSA spends more time reviewing the application and, often, has more documentation of the injury. Still, most survivors are denied benefits a second time. Despite the rash of debilitating brain injuries among our troops in Afghanistan and Iraq, the lifelong, disabling consequences of a brain injury still are underestimated by the Social Security Administration.

As expected, Jessica's request for reconsideration was denied.

Please, don't be discouraged by this second denial. Don't give up. Request a hearing—the next stage in the SSDI appeals process—within sixty days. Then, be prepared for a long wait. In 2007, the average waiting period for a hearing was 520 days. In certain areas, the wait was 900 days.

At the hearing stage, an administrative law judge examines your survivor's application in detail. The hearing is an informal question and answer session held in a closed courtroom. The majority of brain injury SSDI cases are approved at this time.

In Jessica's case, a hearing was scheduled. The judge, however, after reviewing her file prior to the hearing, ruled that there was sufficient documentation to approve her application. A hearing was not necessary.

At any point in this process, you have the right to hire an attorney or someone else to represent you with the Social Security Administration. At the hearing stage, about fifty percent of claimants hire a lawyer to argue their case.

Trying SSDI claims can be a lucrative legal profession. Certain lawyers choose to represent only the best-qualified applicants. In 2009, attorneys were permitted to bill their clients up to $5,300 for a positive outcome. The lawyer collects her fee from your first SSDI payment, which, as noted above, will be a big one.

One way to locate an attorney to represent your survivor is to contact the National Organization of Social Security Claimants' Representatives (800-431-2804 & www.nosscr.org). Also, see the discussion on hiring an attorney on page 139.

If you have patience, excellent communication skills, fine attention to detail, and time, you should be able to represent your patient and save some money. But, it's a gamble I wasn't willing to take when I applied for SSDI for myself eighteen months before Jessica's accident.

If an administrative law judge denies your appeal, you may file a suit in District Court. This court, though, rarely overrules SSA decisions, and it's difficult to find an attorney to represent you at this stage.

Finally, if your application for SSDI is dragging and you are in desperate financial straits, you can try contacting your congressional representatives in Washington, D.C. When I worked for the federal government, I sometimes found a bright red folder, known as a "congressional," in my mail. I was required to respond to this request from a member of Congress for action or information within forty-eight hours. A "congressional" sent to the SSA on behalf of your survivor may speed things up.

Supplemental Security Income

Supplemental Security Income (SSI) is a federal and state government needs-based income program for the aged, blind, and disabled who have limited income and few financial assets.

Here's what you need to know about Supplemental Security Income:

- If your survivor does not qualify for Social Security Disability Income (SSDI), she may be eligible for SSI.

- SSI is funded by federal and state tax revenues.

- The federal portion of SSI is administered by the SSA (800-772-1213 & www.ssa.gov/disability).

131

- Some states supplement the federal benefit.

- SSI has strict eligibility rules. If you think your survivor may qualify, contact the Social Security Administration.

- The monthly SSI benefit varies among states and is based on the recipient's living arrangement and other income, including earnings from work, Social Security and other government benefits, child support, and gifts of food, clothing, or shelter.

- People who qualify for SSI usually are also eligible for food stamps and Medicaid (see page 120).

Workers' Compensation

Workers' Compensation is a state-mandated medical, disability, and life insurance program for people injured on the job. If your survivor was hurt at work, this is what you need to know about Workers' Compensation:

- Most employers must have Workers' Comp insurance.

- Workers' Comp laws are complex and vary from state to state.

- In some states, public funds are used when an injured worker is employed by an uninsured company.

- The claimant usually is sent to a doctor recruited and paid for by her employer.

- If the claimant is temporarily unable to work, she usually will collect two-thirds of her wages up to a fixed ceiling.

- If the claimant is permanently unable to perform her job or work at all, she may be eligible for long-term or lump-sum benefits. The payment amount depends on the nature and extent of her injury.

- In exchange for these guaranteed disability benefits, the claimant usually does not have the right to sue her employer.

- However, if your patient was hurt because of reckless or calculated action by her employer, she can bypass the Workers' Compensation system and sue in court for a full range of damages.

- To know your rights, pick up a copy of the rules in your state from its Workers' Compensation office (see the blue pages in your phone book).

- There may be a time limit for filing a Workers' Comp claim.

- Employers sometimes vigorously contest employee claims.

- If this happens, consult a lawyer with experience handling Workers' Compensation claims on behalf of injured workers.

- Laws in many states limit legal fees to a certain fraction of the award (ten to forty percent). You pay only if you win the case.

- In most cases, jurisdiction over Workers' Compensation disputes is handled by an administrative law judge.

- Appeals may be taken to the court system, but such appeals are viewed skeptically by state appellate courts.

- The Workers' Comp system sometimes provides vocational rehabilitation benefits, such as on-the-job training, schooling, and/or job placement assistance.

Disability Pay & Health Insurance for Children

If your survivor is under the age of eighteen, she may be eligible for federal and/or state government disability pay and health insurance programs. There are a number of these programs and locating the appropriate one for your child might take some legwork. Here are some details to get you started.

Supplemental Security Income for Children

Children who are under the age of eighteen and come from low income families may be eligible for Supplemental Security Income (SSI). Here's what you need to know:

- Children with a brain injury will qualify for Supplemental Security Income if they meet the following two requirements:

  1. They are disabled as defined by the Social Security Administration definition of disability for children.

2. The income and resources of both the child and the family members fall within the eligibility limits.

- To meet the Social Security Administration definition of disability, the child must satisfy the following three requirements:

  1. The child must not be working and earning more than $980 a month in 2009.

  2. The child must have a physical or mental condition or a combination of conditions that result in "marked and severe functional limitations." This means that the child must be severely limited by her medical condition(s).

  3. The child's condition must have lasted, or be expected to last, at least twelve months; or be expected to result in death.

- The amount of the SSI payment is different from one state to another because some states add to the SSI payment.

- If a child is in a medical facility and health insurance pays for her care, the monthly payment in 2009 is limited to $30.

- If the SSA cannot make a disability decision using the medical information, school records, and other facts they have collected, they may send the child for a medical exam, at their cost.

- It can take three to five months for the Social Security Administration to decide if your child is disabled. However, they consider some medical conditions so severe they will begin making payments immediately and for up to six months while they decide if the child is, indeed, disabled. (Despite numerous telephone calls, I was unable to determine if brain injury is one of these conditions.)

- In the Supplemental Security Income program, a child becomes an adult at age eighteen and is reevaluated within one year following her eighteenth birthday. The Social Security Administration then uses different medical and non-medical rules to determine if the claimant can continue to receive SSI payments. The differences are that:

  o Only the survivor's income and resources are counted, not her parents', and

  o The survivor must be disabled as defined by the disability rules for adults, not children.

- Children who were not eligible due to their parents' income and resources may become eligible for SSI at age eighteen.

- When applying for Supplemental Security Income for your child, you will need records that show your income and financial resources, as well as those of your child. It also is helpful to have any school records and the names and contact information for teachers, day care providers, and family members who can describe your child's abilities and disabilities.

Medicaid for Children

In most states, children who receive Supplemental Security Income (SSI) also qualify for Medicaid. In fact, some disabled children are eligible for Medicaid even if they do not qualify for SSI. It's wise to check with your local Social Security office, your state Medicaid agency, or your state or county social services office for more information.

Children with Special Health Care Needs

When your child receives Supplemental Security Income (SSI), she will be referred to health care facilities that provide services under the *Children with Special Needs Provision of the Social Security Act*. These health services usually are managed by state health agencies. Even if your child does not receive SSI, one of these programs may be available to help you. Local health departments, social service offices, and hospitals should be able to help you contact your local Children with Special Health Care Needs program.

The Children's Health Insurance Program

The Children's Health Insurance Program is a federal and state government partnership which enables states to provide health insurance to children from working families with incomes too high to qualify for Medicaid, but too low to afford private health insurance. The program is available throughout the country. You can get more information at 877-543-7669 and www.insurekidsnow.gov.

Social Security Disability Income for Children

The Social Security Disability Income (SSDI) program pays benefits to adults who acquired a disability before reaching age twenty-two. The term for this is an SSDI *child's benefit* because it is paid on a parent's Social Security earnings record. Here's what you need to know about this program:

- For a disabled adult to become entitled to a child's SSDI benefit, at least one of her parents:

  o Must be receiving Social Security retirement or disability benefits; or

  o Must have died and worked long enough to qualify for Social Security benefits.

- Child benefits continue as long as the individual remains disabled.

- At age eighteen, the child is evaluated according to the SSDI definition of disability for adults.

- You can apply for Social Security Disability Income for your child by calling the Social Security Administration (SSA) at 800-772-1213 or by visiting your local Social Security Administration office. You will need your child's birth certificate and Social Security number.

- To expedite the evaluation process, it's best to provide the SSA with as much documentation of your survivor's disability as possible, including the number and dates of hospitalizations, doctor visits, therapy sessions, and copies of any medical records in your possession.

Do We Need an Attorney?

You're exhausted and confused. Your nerves are frazzled. Your medical bills are skyrocketing with no end in sight. You have no idea whether your survivor will ever be able to return to school or work. She may require long-term medical and custodial care. Your financial future may be in jeopardy. But right now you don't want to face these concerns. You just want to be at your survivor's bedside.

An attorney can sort through the complex and time-consuming maze of financial, insurance, and legal matters you're about to encounter.

If there's the possibility of a lawsuit—for or against your loved one—this question is easy to answer. You need an attorney now. Your lawyer will gather evidence about the events causing the injury; collect police reports, photographs, and witness testimony; establish legal responsibility and monetary damages; and try the case.

If your survivor was injured due to the negligence of others, she may be compensated in a court of law for her medical and rehabilitation expenses, loss of income, pain, and suffering.

Otherwise, the decision to hire an attorney demands some thought. Let's consider your situation.

First, you're facing an intimidating pile of paperwork and rounds of trench warfare with your health insurance company and, possibly, your Workers' Compensation, automobile, homeowners, long-term care, and umbrella insurers. They will be looking to minimize their liability. You must be prepared to fight for your rights.

Second, if your survivor is employed, you must file for disability benefits with her employer, any private disability insurance she may have, and with the Social Security Administration. These folks will be in no rush to write you a check.

139

Third, if your patient is older than eighteen years of age and unable to make medical, financial, and legal decisions for herself, you must get permission from the courts to make these decisions for her. Neither a spouse nor a parent automatically becomes the guardian of an incapacitated adult.

Fourth, you may need to arrange for the long-term care of your survivor who may outlive you by decades. This includes estate planning and a special-needs trust.

Many of these crucial matters must be dealt with quickly. They all must be handled accurately.

I chose to handle these matters myself. I had certain advantages. We had great health insurance. I was a career federal government employee with years of experience with arcane regulations, red tape, mountains of paperwork, and bureaucratic trench warfare. Handling these chores gave me a sense of accomplishment when I otherwise felt powerless to help Jessica. The paperwork distracted me from the panic and grief I was trying to contain. Plus, I was fortunate to have people willing to spend time with Jessica when I was filling out forms and making phone calls.

However, I often worried that I would overlook something crucial or make a mistake that we would regret later.

Hiring a competent attorney will give you the peace of mind that these matters are being handled well. It also will eliminate a potentially huge source of stress in an already nerve-wracking time. Best of all, it will give you more time to spend with your survivor, with your family, at your job, or taking care of yourself.

Many of the caregiver panel members hired attorneys and most are glad they did. The downside, of course, is that an attorney will cost you money. If this is an issue, there may be government or nonprofit organizations in your community, such as Legal Aid, that offer free or low-cost legal advice.

Attorneys are compensated in one of two ways: an hourly or pre-determined fee, or a contingency agreement. With a contingency arrangement, the lawyer will represent your survivor for a percentage of the money collected. This enables you to hire an attorney with no money upfront. You pay the lawyer only if you win your case.

If you decide to hire an attorney, keep these guidelines in mind:

- Don't delay, but be deliberate in your choice.

- It's essential that your attorney be intimately familiar with the legal, medical, financial, and long-term issues related to brain injury. The vast majority of lawyers do not have this expertise. Here are four ways to locate attorneys well-versed in brain injury:

  1. Check out the Brain Injury Association of America National Directory of Brain Injury Rehabilitation Services, which includes a list of lawyers throughout the U.S. with experience in brain injury cases (800-444-6443 & www.biausa.org).

  2. Ask your state brain injury association (see page 234) for the names of attorneys who show their interest in brain injury by supporting the association.

  3. Visit the Web site of the American Association for Justice. They have a TBI Litigation Group and a public directory of lawyers who practice in this area (www.justice.org).

  4. Contact your state bar association attorney referral service.

- Interview three or four attorneys. Don't just pick one from the yellow pages, a television commercial, or a billboard.

- Have someone accompany you to the interview to take notes and to provide a second perspective.

- The attorney, not a paralegal (an attorney's assistant), should meet with you in the initial interview.

- Ask for the names and phone numbers of three or four previous clients with brain injuries. Contact them for references.

Here are some more questions to ask in an interview:

- What first interested you in brain injury cases?

- Do you have any special training or education in brain injury law?

- Are you familiar with the long-term challenges of living with a brain injury?

- What local, state, and federal government benefits are my survivor entitled to?

- What experience do you have negotiating with health insurers to obtain benefits for your clients?

- How many brain injury cases have you handled?

- How many trials have you litigated for survivors?

- What were the outcomes of these trials?

- Have you published or lectured in the field of brain injury law?

- Do you attend conferences sponsored by the North American Brain Injury Society, the Brain Injury Association of America, and/or the state brain injury associations?

- How will you determine what impairments my survivor is likely to have?

- How will you educate the judge and jury about these impairments?

- What experts will you retain to help you prepare and try our case?

- Who else in your office will work on our case? What are their credentials?

- Who will be our primary contact?

- How will you calculate the financial settlement we request in the trial?

- How will you help us protect the funds awarded in a settlement or judgment and remain eligible for government benefits, such as Social Security Disability Income, Medicare, and/or Medicaid?

- Is your firm able and willing to advance as much as $50,000 in the investigation, preparation, and presentation of our case?

After the interview, think about how the attorney responded to your questions, how she and the office staff treated you, and how knowledgeable she appeared to be about brain injury. Will you be comfortable working with her, perhaps, for a long time?

Here are four things to keep in mind, when you have selected an attorney to represent your survivor:

1. Be sure you understand and receive in writing your agreement regarding the attorney's fees: the percentage retained in a contingency agreement, the hourly fee in a pay-as-you-go arrangement, or the amount of a pre-determined fee, as well as a detailed explanation of any billable expenses.

2. This written agreement also should indicate whether the attorney will advance the expenses of your case, and who, ultimately, is responsible for the case expenses if the case is settled or lost.

3. A paralegal likely will handle your case on a day-to-day basis. Your attorney, however, should respond to your questions and concerns.

4. If you become dissatisfied with your lawyer, you have the right to switch attorneys at any time during your case. States vary in how a discharged attorney is paid.

Not hiring an attorney worked for us; it may not for you. This is a crucial decision that should be well thought out.

Notes

Checklist for Success #3
Paying the Bills

___ Have you considered sending out-of-town family and friends home so they can save precious hours of leave from work to return when you will need their help much more?

___ Have you familiarized yourself with your survivor's health insurance policy to understand what medical and rehabilitation services will and will not be covered? What are the policy's preauthorization requirements, benefit limits, co-pays, restrictions, and reporting requirements?

___ How much rehabilitation—inpatient and outpatient— will your survivor's health insurance cover?

___ If you fear that your survivor's health insurance is lacking, see page 117.

___ Are there any other insurance policies that may help you pay the medical bills: auto, home, umbrella, disability, long-term care, and workers' compensation?

___ Are your survivor's income and financial assets low enough for her to qualify for Medicaid? [See page 120.]

___ Do you know that if your survivor qualifies for Social Security Disability Income [see page 125], she will become eligible for Medicare in two years? [See page 121.]

___ How long will your survivor continue to receive pay checks while she is unable to work? This depends upon her eligibility for:

- Vacation and sick pay [See page 123.]
- Short-term disability benefits
- Long-term disability benefits
- Leave sharing [See page 125.]
- Social Security Disability Income [See page 125.]
- Supplemental Security Income [See page 131.]
- Workers' Compensation [See page 132.]

___ Have you started the very long process of applying for Social Security Disability Income benefits? It's not too early to begin. [See page 125.]

___ Do you know how to appeal your survivor's case for Social Security Disability Income if her application is denied? Most initial applications involving brain injury are rejected. [See page 129.]

___ Are your survivor's income and financial assets low enough for her to qualify for Supplemental Security Income? [See page 131.]

___ If your survivor was injured on the job, are you aware of the benefits she qualifies for under Workers' Compensation health and disability insurance? [See page 132.]

____ If your survivor is a child under the age of 18, are you aware that she may be eligible for the following benefits?

- Supplemental Security Income for Children [See page 134.]
- Medicaid for Children [See page 137.]
- The Children with Special Health Care Needs Program [See page 137.]
- The Children's Health Insurance Program [See page 137.]
- Social Security Disability Income for Children [See page 138.]

____ Have you considered hiring an attorney for any of the following services: [See page 139.]

- Representing your survivor if she was injured due to the negligence of others
- Ensuring that she receives all of the insurance and disability benefits she's entitled to
- Applying for Social Security Disability Income
- Receiving permission from the courts for you to make medical, financial, and legal decisions for your survivor
- Arranging for her long-term care

____ Is it possible your survivor may need to stay in a skilled nursing facility until she's ready for rehabilitation? If so, have you begun researching the local nursing homes? [See page 206.]

11

Trapped in the Fog
From Coma to
Post-Traumatic Amnesia

In the Intermediate Care Unit (IMC), Jessica was placed in a gloomy, double room that barely benefited from the large window next to her bed. A hulking parking garage blocked the sunlight that might have brightened this depressing room.

Jessica's roommate, Jim, was ten days ahead of her in his recovery. Susan and Jim had three teenage daughters who rarely came to the hospital. Susan chose to keep their lives as normal as possible. Caregivers like Susan, like all of us, face a tough decision. How do you spread your limited time and energy among your survivor, your family, and your job, and still have a bit of time for yourself? For the first time, I was glad my disabilities relieved me of the daily grind of work. I was able to be with Jessica every morning and early afternoon before my uncooperative body sent me home.

Jessica's sister Barbara and I now took turns trying to coax Jessica out of her coma. (Yes, we both have sisters named Barbara. Fortunately, their appearances do not overlap in the story.) We sat by Jessica's bed, spoke to her softly, held her

149

hand, cooled her face with a wet cloth, and, at last, saw the first signs of an emerging consciousness.

Jessica opened her eyes briefly. She squeezed our hands. She scratched her nose. She turned her head in the direction of our voices. Dr. Thomas and the nurses were quick to warn us that these actions were involuntary neurological responses, not the purposeful acts that signal the end of a coma. Despite this explanation, we couldn't help but view them with hope and joy.

Jessica clearly was reacting to her pain as her fractured bones and pummeled internal organs slowly healed. When a nurse drew blood gases, Jessica recoiled from the sting. She occasionally became agitated, tossing and turning, trying, in our minds, to find relief from her unrelenting pain. Her pulse and blood pressure sometimes soared; she required coma-extending sedatives to calm her.

Two weeks after her accident, Jessica opened her eyes and, for the first time, she kept them open. She scanned the room for twenty seconds and then slipped back into her slumber. Over the next few hours, she followed this pattern. Once, she seemed to examine the splint on her right arm and hand. Five minutes later, she tried to remove her thumb from the splint.

Within two days, Jessica was opening her eyes at my request and reaching for my hand. I believe she tried to speak, and I thought I saw tears well up in her eyes. When I bent down to hug her, she sometimes rubbed my back in a reassuring manner. Her sister Barbara and I were thrilled.

I reported these momentous events to Dr. Thomas whenever he stopped by. But, he remained skeptical; Jessica wouldn't respond to his commands.

In a way, Jessica was doing just fine in practice with me coaching her through every step of emerging from a coma. She couldn't produce at game time, however, in front of a crowd, a.k.a. the Chief of Trauma Services.

Jessica's time in the IMC was the beginning of two weeks of torment for both of us. So far, I had just seen Jessica resting quietly with a few distressing, but brief, demonstrations of pain and bewilderment. This was about to change. Despite all my reading, I was ill-prepared for what happened next.

First, a new player entered the picture. Dr. Stevens was the *physiatrist* (a doctor who specializes in rehabilitation) treating Jessica. To our relief, he agreed with our assessment of Jessica's condition. "She's improving," he said. "Dr. Thomas is just being guarded. That's the way he is."

Jessica was transitioning from coma to *post-traumatic amnesia*, a time of bafflement and agitation nearly all survivors pass through on their way back to full consciousness. For the next two weeks, Jessica was in the worst state imaginable. When awake, she was constantly moving, thrashing about her bed like a terrified, wounded beast. She was panicked, frustrated, and combative. She persistently tried to pull the ventilator tube out of her tracheotomy. She struggled to climb out of bed, jeopardizing her still unmended bones.

Jessica resisted all our efforts to calm her. We were unable to communicate with her. She had no concept of language. She was acting instinctively, rebelling against her pain and perplexity in a primitive, inhuman manner. I had to restrain her arms and legs whenever I left her alone, which made both of us miserable.

Fortunately, Jessica has no memory of this time. For those of us at her bedside, it was agonizing. I knew this was a normal stage of recovery. It was hard to believe, however, that Jessica would ever progress beyond this helpless, distraught, unaware condition to someone who even remotely resembled her old self.

Many times, I was desperate to flee her room. One day, our friend Pat was scheduled to sit with Jessica while I ate lunch. The last time Pat had seen Jessica, she was lying quietly in a coma. Pat was totally unprepared for this new, restless, anguished Jessica.

Pat was running late; I was boiling over. When she finally arrived, I managed a quick hello and bolted from the room, unforgivably leaving Pat and Jessica to fend for themselves.

Jessica's Aunt Anita had the bad luck to be helping us during the first week of Jessica's post-traumatic amnesia. Anita had traveled north from Florida to spend time with Jessica and to keep me well fed. She returned home convinced that Jessica would never be able to care for herself or even be left unattended. Anita feared that my expectations for Jessica's recovery were far from realistic. She was certain I was in for a terrible shock when I ultimately recognized Jessica's true condition.

Weeks later, when Jessica was about halfway through her inpatient rehabilitation, she made her first phone call. At the other end of the line, her aunt was delightfully shocked to hear Jessica say "Hello Anita."

From my reading and fleeting conversations with Dr. Thomas, I knew that the support of family and friends during rehabilitation motivates the patient to work harder and recover more successfully. Given my physical limitations, I couldn't provide all of the support Jessica would need in the coming months. I realized that I needed someone at the house to assist me with the chores and to be with Jessica in the late afternoon and early evening.

My first thought was to recruit one of Jessica's six siblings to put his or her life on hold for a few months and help me care for Jessica. I soon realized this was asking a lot.

They had young children to raise and jobs and school to manage. So, I broadcast my need for support to our growing email list of family and friends. I hoped some folks would be willing and able to give us a week of their time. A few days would be nice, but not as helpful. It took time to adjust to Jessica's condition to be an effective caregiver.

The response was remarkable. I was able to schedule a helper—a sister, a brother, a parent, an aunt, a friend, or a cousin—staying at the house with me for many weeks.

I don't know what I would have done without these folks. I couldn't spend all day with Jessica and she would have suffered, restrained in her bed, alone with her pain and disorientation. I might have pushed myself too hard, perhaps ending up in bed myself. I also would have felt abandoned in the most trying time of my life. Even an introvert sometimes yearns for the company of others. I also needed the reassurance from my houseguests that I was managing Jessica's care as well as possible, because I had plenty of doubts.

Jessica had a parade of visitors, particularly on weekends. Certain people just knew how to be helpful. A coworker stopped by for just five minutes to let me know she was thinking about us. She also brought the unlikely gift of smoked salmon, knowing that it's one of my favorite foods. Perfect.

Other people had no clue. They were uneasy and didn't know what to say. Some tried to hide their nervousness with small talk; others tossed out exasperating clichés.

She's lucky to be alive.

She'll be better in no time.

This whole experience will make the two of you stronger.

Some visitors stayed well beyond their welcome. If they were intent on remaining, I could have used the opportunity to get some fresh air or relax my guard for a few minutes. But, I was comfortable leaving Jessica alone with only a handful of people. The others appeared too shaken to be useful. After too many awkward visits, I asked most people to stay away until Jessica was more coherent and less frantic.

Adding to Jessica's peculiar behavior was an out-of-whack internal thermostat, a typical problem with brain injury. Jessica was unbearably warm, and lacking any shame, she instinctually shed her clothing, every bit of her clothing. After seeing this twice, Anita fashioned a modesty tent with a pair of bed sheets, allowing Jessica to be cool while maintaining her dignity.

Anita also rescued Jessica from my periodic lapses of common sense. For example, it didn't occur to me to untangle the knots in Jessica's long hair as she lay in bed day after day. By the time Anita spotted the problem, it was too late. The only solution was to start cutting. Jessica didn't appreciate this when she began to recognize herself in a mirror.

While Dr. Thomas remained cautious with his diagnosis, Dr. Stevens agreed with us that Jessica had graduated to *Level 3: Localized Response* on the Rancho Scale. He believed she was ready to benefit from rehabilitation.

> **Level 3: Localized Response.** The patient reacts more appropriately, but still inconsistently, to stimuli, especially bright light, sound, and physical discomfort. She inconsistently follows simple commands, such as "Close your eyes" or "Squeeze my hand." She may occasionally turn her head in the direction of a speaker's voice.

Jessica kept her eyes open more each day. I was confident that when she slept, she would wake up when I talked to her. She seemed to recognize me—maybe not as her husband—but as a good guy in a world filled with bad guys. In those infrequent moments when she was calm, she stroked my back, scratched my beard, and reached for my hand. Then a fury of pain, perplexity, and frustration would overtake her.

Positive things were happening. Jessica's breathing had stabilized; she was being weaned off the ventilator. She was yawning and coughing, and, I thought, trying to speak, which was impossible with the ventilator tube in her windpipe. Her temperature dropped to near normal; the threat of a major infection was over. She was sitting in a more upright position twice a day, slowly regaining some strength.

Of course, the negatives still far outweighed the positives. Jessica's latest MRI showed a blood clot and continued swelling in her brain, which could create major problems with her rehabilitation. Plus, we were far from knowing which life-altering impairments we would have to confront thanks to Jessica's moment of inattentive driving.

Survivors of not-so-serious brain injuries often go straight home from the emergency room or the hospital with, maybe, some outpatient rehabilitation. For most survivors with serious injuries, the next stop is either an inpatient rehabilitation facility or a nursing home. At this stage in their recovery, they generally need too much skilled medical attention to be cared for at home.

The choice between a rehab facility and a nursing home is based on the patient's ability to participate in rehabilitation as measured by the Rancho Scale. Three parties have a say in this decision: (1) the trauma doctor, (2) the rehabilitation facility, and (3) the health insurer.

Jessica's condition now was becoming too stable for acute care. In Dr. Thomas's eyes, however, she wasn't ready for rehab. Plus, our health insurer would not pay for inpatient rehab until Jessica reached *Level 4*. Though, the rehabilitation facility was willing to admit her at *Level 3*. It was a predicament.

We faced the unhappy prospect of transferring Jessica to a nursing home. Dr. Thomas's caution worried us. So, we began to try to muster the thousands of dollars needed to pay for a week or two of inpatient rehabilitation ourselves.

Notes

12

Life with a Brain Injury Preparing Yourself and Your Family

The brain oversees everything we do:

- How we move our body (physical)
- How we perceive, recall, and process information (cognitive)
- How we communicate with others (communication)
- How we feel (emotional)
- How we behave (behavioral)
- How we interact with others (social)

It's easy to see how a serious blow to the brain can have a devastating impact on the survivor and those around her.

As different parts of the brain control different functions, the impairments acquired by a survivor depend on the precise location and gravity of her injury. Since every injury is unique in the damage it causes, every survivor acquires a unique mix of complaints.

It's impossible for a doctor to review your patient's CT scans and MRIs and predict the deficits she will acquire. Certain functions, however, such as memory, language, and information processing, are lodged in multiple areas of the brain and are almost always affected by any serious injury.

Later in this section, I list the more common impairments of a serious brain injury, divided into the six categories described above. As you review these lists, remember, no one survivor will experience all of these complaints.

There is a powerful cause and effect relationship among the impairments produced by a brain injury. Some can be called *primary*; others can be called *secondary*.

Primary impairments are those directly related to brain damage. These include most of the complaints in the physical and cognitive categories. Secondary impairments are those that develop as a consequence of one or more primary impairments. Communication and social complaints mostly are secondary impairments. Emotional and behavioral complaints generally occur as both primary and secondary impairments.

This can be confusing. So, let's consider five examples:

1. Mary was a marathon runner; she now walks with a distinct shuffle (primary physical). This humiliates her (secondary emotional). So she rarely leaves her house (secondary behavioral and social).

2. Susan was training to be a doctor. Her injury dashed her dream (primary cognitive). She is now depressed (secondary emotional) and not much fun to be around (secondary social).

3. Changes in the chemistry of Beth's brain cause her to be jittery (primary emotional). Medication helps, but the drugs cloud her already foggy thinking (secondary cognitive). She gulps Mylanta to quell her anxiety-driven heartburn (secondary physical).

4. Nancy was an auctioneer. She now has a problem expressing herself (primary physical and cognitive, and secondary communication). She lost her job and is worried about paying the rent (secondary emotional). Her anxiety causes her to unconsciously tense her muscles, aggravating the pain in her spastic arm (secondary physical).

5. Martha's major complaints are disinhibition (primary behavioral) and impaired short-term memory (primary cognitive). She's the life of the party. But, she lost her job as a waitress because she spent too much time flirting with the customers (secondary social) and mixed up her orders too often (secondary communication).

It is important to understand that secondary impairments can be just as debilitating as primary impairments.

Warning: Some caregivers tell me they preferred not to know what the ultimate outcome might be for their survivor. Others, like me, wanted to know all the possibilities right away: the worst case, the best case, and everything in between. If you'd rather not speculate about the future, that's okay. Just jump to the next section.

Physical Impairments

Physical complaints are the easiest to detect and the quickest to be treated. There's no hiding that somebody walks with a shuffle or has little coordination in her left extremities. While many physical deficits are permanent, others can be remedied or moderated with physical therapy and other types of treatment, such as exercise, surgery, and prescription medication, taken orally or injected into troublesome areas.

The one physical complaint every survivor experiences is fatigue, particularly during the early days of recovery and rehabilitation. The healing brain devours energy. The patient's remaining get-up-and-go is gone quickly. The injured brain must work double-, triple-, or even quadruple-time to perform even simple tasks. In rehab, Jessica sometimes slept sixteen or more hours a day. Even today, she frequently needs eleven or twelve hours of sleep to re-energize herself.

Some of the other typical physical complaints caused by a brain injury are:

- Headaches
- Spasticity
- Partial paralysis
- Seizures
- Chronic pain
- Disturbed sleep
- Poor endurance
- Speech difficulties
- Swallowing difficulties
- Changes in appetite
- Hypersensitivity
- Muscle weakness
- Altered sexual response
- Changes in appearance

Also, it's not uncommon for survivors to find one or more of their senses—sight, hearing, touch, taste, and smell—altered by their injury.

Finally, many folks living with brain injury are clumsy due to impaired muscle coordination, balance, and motor control.

Cognitive Impairments

Cognitive complaints, almost always, are the most disabling of the six types of impairments caused by a brain injury. They are most profound immediately after the injury when the survivor has very limited awareness.

During rehabilitation, cognitive abilities typically improve dramatically, but rarely fully. All but a handful of survivors of serious brain injuries experience major cognitive deficits.

In the past, it was believed that, after two years, people living with a brain injury made little or no progress in cognitive ability. New research, however, has demonstrated that recovery can, with effort, be a lifelong exercise.

Cognitive impairments—by themselves or in combination—cause many problems in daily life. Take reading, for example. One person has difficulty reading because her injury damaged the language centers of her brain. She can't comprehend the meaning of many words. A second person struggles to read since her injury compromised her short-term memory. She can't follow the flow of a story. A third cancelled her library card because her injury ravaged her ability to concentrate. She started a book twenty times and never got past the first page.

Neuropsychological testing is a tool rehabilitation therapists use to isolate the cognitive impairments—such as language, memory, and/or concentration—that cause a particular functional problem, such as difficulty reading.

Unlike physical complaints, which are easily diagnosed, cognitive impairments can be subtle. This is especially true with a package of higher-level cognitive abilities called *executive functioning*. We use our executive functioning abilities to do everything from making an egg salad sandwich to launching a spacecraft. The survivor and those around her often don't recognize major deficits in this area until she returns home and reenters the community.

Memory almost always is impaired by a brain injury. Four types of memory can be affected, singly or in combination:

1. Short-term: the ability to hold a small amount of information for about twenty seconds
2. Long-term: the ability to hold and retrieve information for as little as a few days and as long as a few decades
3. Retrograde: the ability to recall events that occurred prior to the injury
4. Anterograde: the ability to recall events that occurred after the injury

The most debilitating cognitive complaint is a lack of awareness of one's deficits. Without this realization, the survivor sees no reason to work hard to recover her cognitive abilities and, thereby, remains seriously impaired. She may become belligerent as she is unable to understand why her life has become so difficult.

Other common cognitive complaints include deficits in the following areas:

- Attention
- Comprehension
- Concentration
- Decision-making
- Initiation
- Judgment
- Self-monitoring
- Spatial orientation
- Language comprehension
- Safety awareness
- Information processing
- Learning new material

You may find that your survivor dresses in the morning before showering or is overwhelmed at the idea of preparing a simple lunch of soup and a sandwich. Her executive functioning abilities have been disturbed by her brain injury. These are the primary components of executive-functioning:

- Analyzing
- Prioritizing
- Planning
- Sequencing
- Organizing
- Directing
- Multi-tasking
- Monitoring
- Reasoning
- Evaluating
- Troubleshooting
- Problem-solving

Two common, but usually temporary, cognitive complaints are *confabulation* and *perseveration*. Confabulation, also known as false memory, is the confusion of imagination and memory. The patient, struggling to explain the gaps in her memory and her bewilderment and fear as she emerges from her coma, creates a, sometimes, bizarre fantasy. She doesn't grasp that she has been injured and is in a hospital. Some survivors actually believe they are being held prisoner and are the subjects of strange experiments or sadistic behaviors.

Perseveration is the persistent repetition of a response—a word, a phrase, or a gesture, when the stimulus that triggered the response has disappeared. For example, the patient may respond to a question and then repeat the answer over and over, even well after the person who posed the question has left the room.

Communication Impairments

Physical and cognitive complaints routinely impair a survivor's ability to communicate. The physical impediments include:

- Illegible handwriting
- Painfully slow handwriting
- Slurred speech
- Speaking too slowly or too quickly
- Speaking too loudly or too softly
- Impaired hearing and/or sight
- Impaired verbal fluency

The cognitive impediments to communication include:

- Inability to understand words
- Reading impairment
- Difficulty finding words
- Difficulty expressing ideas
- Verbal disinhibition
- Difficulty getting to the point
- Poor listening attention

Emotional Impairments

Emotional complaints arise either directly from the injury to the brain or indirectly as a reaction to one or more primary impairments. For example, one survivor is depressed due to damage to the part of the brain that governs emotions. A second survivor is depressed because she has trouble expressing herself and has lost nearly all her friends.

Often, when a patient slowly regains consciousness, she is in a pleasant mood as her view of the world clears. Later, when she begins to recognize the extent of her impairments, she becomes vulnerable to a wide range of debilitating emotions. These emotions can be treated—with full or partial effectiveness—through individual or group therapy, peer counseling, help from a support group, and/or medication.

The more common emotional complaints caused by a brain injury are:

- Anger
- Anxiety
- Apathy
- Confusion
- Denial
- Depression
- Egocentricity
- Embarrassment
- Frustration
- Irritability
- Mood swings
- Paranoia
- Post-traumatic stress
- Psychosomatic pain
- Restlessness
- Self-esteem loss
- Self-hatred
- Stubbornness

Behavioral Impairments

As with emotional complaints, behavioral problems result from a combination of direct and indirect causes. Damage to the area of the brain that houses self-control and social awareness can rob the survivor of the filter that keeps her behavior consistent with socially accepted norms.

One survivor may throw a temper tantrum at the grocery store because she can't find those last two items on her shopping list, and she is too tired to monitor her own behavior. Another survivor may act up in a movie theater because she can't follow the plot of the film and doesn't recognize that her fidgeting and complaining is annoying people sitting nearby.

Behavioral complaints, which can interfere with rehabilitation, range from simply annoying to the threat of bodily harm to the survivor and/or the people around her.

The more common behavioral complaints caused by a brain injury are:

- Alcohol abuse
- Clinging
- Complaining
- Crying excessively
- Cursing
- Defensiveness
- Destructiveness
- Disinhibition
- Immaturity
- Impulsivity
- Inflexibility

- Intolerance
- Overreaction
- Paranoia
- Physical aggression
- Rebelliousness
- Selfishness
- Sexual inappropriateness
- Sexual promiscuity
- Under-reaction
- Verbal aggression
- Withdrawal

Sometimes, behavioral problems don't develop until the survivor returns home and expects her life to return to normal. They also can undermine a survivor's transition back into the community.

Behavioral problems can be tricky to treat and require considerable patience and understanding from others. Extreme behavioral impairments require highly structured treatment by professionals in an inpatient setting.

Social Impairments

Probably the most common social complaint arising from a brain injury is loneliness. It's easy to imagine how a mix of physical, cognitive, communication, emotional, and behavioral problems can scare away old friends and frustrate finding new ones. This is particularly true among the largest group of survivors, young men just entering adulthood. Their buddies are quick to move on when their pal can't keep up with them. Many survivors rely heavily on their families to satisfy their social needs.

Brain injury also is cruel to romantic relationships, especially newer ones. "You're not the same person I fell in love with," is heard frequently by people with a brain injury. Some survivors become self-centered and unable to recognize and respond to the needs of their partners. Some partners are unwilling to adjust to the transformation in their survivors.

In a culture influenced heavily by the beauty and witty repartee of television and film stars, many people discount the possibility of becoming friends with someone who has multiple impairments. This unfortunate bias limits a survivor's chances to meet new people, especially those looking for romance.

Despite these obstacles, however, plenty of survivors on the panel remain happily married. Others have discovered love and marriage after their brain injury.

These are the primary complaints that create social barriers for survivors:

- Visible physical impairments which make some people uncomfortable
- Fatigue that limits social activities
- Difficulty finding words in conversation
- Difficulty interpreting customary social cues
- Unemployment, which reduces social opportunities

- An inability to drive or use public transportation, which keeps survivors at home
- Emotional problems, such as anger, apathy, denial, depression, egocentricity, and paranoia
- Behavioral problems, such as aggression, complaining, destructiveness, immaturity, selfishness, and withdrawal

Spasticity

Spasticity is a condition of abnormally increased muscle tone or the shortening and/or tightening of soft tissue muscles, tendons, and ligaments. A common symptom of serious brain injuries, spasticity is caused by damage to a particular part of the brain or tears in the bundles of nerves around the brainstem that control movement and sensation.

To appreciate what a spastic muscle feels like, concentrate on one of your muscles. Tense this muscle as if it's being worked to its limit. Then, try to imagine how you would go about your daily activities with this muscle permanently contracted.

A posture characteristic of spasticity is legs stretched out straight and stiff and arms bent up at the elbow. Other areas commonly affected by spasticity are the shoulders, elbows, wrists, fists, thumbs, feet, toes, knees, thighs, and hips.

The principal characteristics of spasticity are:

- Extreme muscle tightness and spasms
- Physical deformity or abnormal posture
- Restricted movements
- Pain, possibly extreme, potentially leading to secondary spasticity
- Potential dislocation of a joint or organ
- Skin ulcers

- Functional limitations, such as

  o The inability to use a hand in daily activities
  o Difficulty with transfers, such as from a car to a wheelchair
  o Impaired gait
  o Impaired speech

The severity of spasticity, which can worsen with time, ranges from mild muscle stiffness to painful, crippling, uncontrollable muscle spasms. Spasticity can be a terrible problem, sometimes interfering with the patient's ability to swallow, eat, speak, and eliminate waste. It also can be a major impediment to rehabilitation. Cold weather, fatigue, and multi-tasking can exacerbate the spasms.

For survivors who have extreme mobility impairments, spasticity, at times, can be helpful. Stiffness of the lower limbs can support the individual's weight when transferring or walking.

Often, spasticity resolves with time and therapy, although it may never disappear. A combination of treatments is used to prevent the further shortening of muscles and to reduce the severity of the symptoms:

- Daily exercise, including sustained stretching and range-of-motion movements
- Electrical muscle stimulation
- Orthotics
- Casts or braces
- Surgery to release tendons or to block the connection between nerve and muscle
- Oral medication, which can result in sedation, weakness, and cognitive impairment

- Injected medication, which can temporarily block the connection between nerve and muscle, but it has unpleasant side effects and can become less potent with time
- A baclofen pump, which, when implanted into the body and programmed to dispense medication, can reduce spasms. A pump demands a considerable commitment of time and attention by both survivor and caregiver.

Seizures

Seizures or post-traumatic epilepsy also occur sometimes after a brain injury.

For decades researchers believed that seizures were caused by sudden and unpredictable abnormal electrical activity in the brain. New research suggests that chemicals released by the brain itself, in an effort to repair the injured site, may be the cause.

The symptoms of post-traumatic epilepsy depend on where in the brain the abnormality (electrical or chemical) occurs. Seizures can be confined to a small area or involve the entire brain. Their severity ranges from mild discomfort and disorientation to extreme physical and mental disability. Seizures can last from a few seconds to five minutes.

About ten percent of survivors develop post-traumatic epilepsy and experience continuing seizures. Patients with scarring on the brain from skull fractures, penetrating injuries, bruising, and focal bleeding, are at the greatest risk of having seizures.

A brain injury survivor usually will have her first seizure soon after her injury. The first seizure, however, can occur as much as four to twenty years after the injury, depending on which research you read.

A seizure can be a one-time event or a lifelong problem. Jessica had a seizure in the emergency room soon after her accident, but none since.

Most post-traumatic epilepsy responds well to anti-convulsant medications. Finding the best drug and dosage, however, can take time, and anti-convulsants can trigger unpleasant side-effects. Taking medication, however, is essential. Uncontrolled seizures can further damage the brain.

The symptoms of post-traumatic epilepsy can be subtle to extreme. They vary widely among people.

The subtle symptoms, which are known collectively as an *aura,* include the following:

- A momentary disturbance in attention
- A brief period of restlessness or disorientation
- Sudden and unexplainable feelings of fear, anger, sadness, and/or nausea
- An altered sense of hearing, smell, taste, sight, and/or touch
- A feeling of being detached from the environment
- Déjà vu (familiarity) or jamais vu (unfamiliarity)
- Labored speech or the inability to speak
- Brief loss of memory

In more serious cases, after experiencing an aura, a person might:

- Stare into space or have a blank look
- Be confused, unresponsive, and unaware of her surroundings
- Act strangely by smacking her lips, swallowing, chewing, picking at her clothing, or wandering
- Not recall the seizure afterward

With the most severe seizures, the person might exhibit the following symptoms:

- Fall to the ground
- Convulse violently with stiff and jerking movements
- Moan
- Breathe shallowly or stop breathing momentarily
- Roll back her eyes
- Bite her tongue
- Lose bladder or bowel control

Given these symptoms, persons prone to seizures must avoid situations that can place themselves or somebody else at risk. Driving is the most inconvenient of these restrictions, which also include using power tools, climbing ladders, and swimming and bathing alone.

The Impact of Brain Injury on the Family

A brain injury places enormous stress on the survivor's family. In the first days or weeks, the family is in crisis mode. Day-to-day routines and the needs of other members are cast aside as the family spends hours at the hospital. The focus of attention is on the patient. Everyone is battered by a wide range of emotions: worry, guilt, anger, helplessness, and grief, among others. Later, when the survivor returns home, each family member must learn to accommodate her impairments, adjust to new routines, and, possibly, assume new roles and responsibilities within the household.

There is no single correct way a family should act immediately after a brain injury. Some people are at ease and useful at the hospital. Others are too traumatized to approach the patient. Some people will spend most of their time at the

171

hospital. Others will return to work or school, by choice or necessity. Everyone must adjust in his own way and at his own pace.

The circumstances of the injury may create tension. There may be guilt ("Why did I allow her to buy a motorcycle?") or accusation ("Why weren't you watching her?").

If the survivor contributed to her injury, there may be anger ("How many times did I tell her to buckle her seat belt?").

Issues among family members, unresolved before the injury, may explode under the stress of the situation. The strength and harmony of the family will be tested by the uncertainty of the survivor's outcome:

- How well will the patient recover?
- How will an incomplete recovery impact the dynamics of the family?
- How much will the medical costs and possible loss of the survivor's income upset the family budget?
- How will the family cope as members assume new and unfamiliar responsibilities?
- How will the family manage when everyone returns to their own lives at school, at work, and in the community, but also must care for the survivor?

These tensions can be heightened if the patient is hospitalized far from home. The caregiver can feel imprisoned in a disagreeable hospital setting, lonely and isolated from family and friends, and guilty for not tending to responsibilities at home. The folks at home may suffer from the absence of two family members, especially if it is both parents.

Later, the family may feel isolated when the immediate crisis passes and relatives and friends return to their own busy lives and provide less support.

Adult children, who live away from home, might be torn between two families. They dearly want to help care for their injured sister, but they have more pressing obligations to their spouse, children, and employer.

Jessica and I have no children and I was retired at the time of her collision. So, I was able to focus my time and energy on her recovery and rehabilitation.

Most of the caregivers on the panel, however, were forced to juggle caring for their survivor, their children, their job, and other responsibilities. I have relied heavily on their input to offer the following advice for parents trying to cope with a brain injury in the family.

Coping with Emotions

A brain injury places great stress on every member of the household. If this stress is not addressed, it can tear a family apart. Your children will look to you as a guide, seeing from your words and behavior the gravity of the situation.

Here are nine suggestions for defusing emotional landmines before they explode:

1. In general, be calm and in control.
2. But, at times, show your emotions. This will tell your children that the emotions they are feeling are natural.
3. Discuss your emotions with your children.
4. Encourage them to talk about their feelings.
5. Don't give them the impression you expect them to be brave and not show their sadness.
6. Listen carefully. Your children may talk about their emotions in a roundabout manner.
7. Be careful with older children. Teenagers may appear strong and in control but be hurting desperately inside.

8. If you sense a decline in the emotional health of your family, pick up a copy of *Missing Pieces: Mending the Head Injury Family* by Marilyn Colter, a journalist, mother, and insightful caregiver of her husband, a brain injury survivor. (See page 232.)
9. If emotions are running wild, it's probably time to consult a professional counselor.

Caring for Young Children

It's understandable that you will concentrate your time and energy on your patient and will spend many hours at the hospital. It's crucial, however, that other family members—especially young children—don't feel forgotten. Here are nine ways to keep young children feeling loved and well cared for:

1. For nearly all children, trying to keep their lives as normal as possible is the best advice.
2. Help them stay in touch with friends.
3. Be sure they have their usual enjoyable activities.
4. Settle your children back into their normal school routine and inform their principal of the situation.
5. Set aside one-on-one time with your children when you are home.
6. If you can't be home, set a time for a daily phone call to catch up with the latest news in their lives.
7. Have somebody drive your children to their favorite activities. Try not to let these activities lapse.
8. Ask somebody to relieve you at the hospital to allow you some quality time with your children.
9. Don't be surprised if the behavior of your children regresses as they compete for your attention.

What Do I Tell My Children?

You are the best judge of how much to tell your children about your survivor's injury. Bear in mind, however, that even the youngest child knows a bad thing has happened and may imagine all sorts of horrors until his questions are answered. Here are ten ways to keep your children informed and prepared for an upheaval in family life and routines:

1. Encourage your children to ask questions. Answer these questions as simply and accurately as you can.
2. Fit your explanations to their level of language, maturity, and comprehension.
3. Use concrete examples: "Your mother may have trouble speaking" or "She will be exhausted when she comes home."
4. When you don't have the answer, admit it. Promise to find the answer.
5. If you're having trouble answering questions, find someone who can.
6. Provide repeated opportunities for children to ask questions and to absorb what's happened.
7. Share new developments, good and bad, as they occur.
8. Avoid well-meaning clichés like "Everything will be all right." With a serious brain injury, everything will not be all right. You don't want to create false hope to be cruelly shattered later.
9. Be sure everyone grasps the gravity of the situation to the best of their ability. This provides time to adjust to the changes in your survivor before she returns home.
10. Your children may have questions they are not comfortable asking you. See if they want to speak to someone else about your family member's injury.

Bringing Children to the Hospital

You also are the best judge of whether your children will benefit from visiting your survivor in the hospital. Here are eight guidelines to keep in mind when weighing the pluses and minuses of a visit:

1. Don't force a child to visit an injured family member.

2. A possible exception to this rule is if the patient is alert and a visit with the child will be therapeutic.

3. Prepare your child for what he will see at the hospital:

   - The patient's appearance and behavior
   - The sounds and smells in her room
   - The wires and lines connected to her
   - The machines surrounding her
   - How he should act with her

4. Let your child choose when and for how long to visit.

5. Tell your child that it's okay to be nervous or scared.

6. Introduce your child to the doctors and nurses. This will give him an opportunity to pose questions to the experts.

7. If he's willing, encourage your child to help care for the patient. This may comfort both parties.

8. If your child doesn't wish to visit, he may feel guilty. Encourage him to participate in caring for your survivor in other ways, such as drawing pictures and sending cards and letters.

Children Growing Up Too Quickly

A brain injury in the family can force your child to grow up too quickly if he's overloaded with new responsibilities. Be careful.

- Don't burden your child with duties far beyond his age.
- Let him know you appreciate the sacrifices he's making to be helpful at home.
- Be sure he keeps up with his school work.
- Don't ask him to be brave beyond his years. Let him grieve, be angry, and act immaturely at times. Venting emotions is an essential aspect of coming to terms with a brain injury.

Giving Older Children a Role

Some older children will want to be involved in their family member's recovery. This should be encouraged to the extent their maturity permits. Others will not. This is okay, but asking them to assume more responsibility at home is reasonable.

Your older child can do some or all of the following:

- Keep a list of questions for the doctors.
- Accompany you when you speak with the physicians.
- Record the doctor's answers to your questions.
- Learn to assist in the care of your patient.
- Sit with your survivor in the hospital.
- Surf the Internet for information about brain injury.
- Write a newsletter or launch a Web site to update family and friends on your survivor's condition.
- Take on more of the household chores and errands.
- Care for younger siblings.

Checklist for Success #4
Preparing Yourself and Your Family

___ Have you decided how you are going to allocate your time among your survivor, your family, your job, and your other responsibilities?

___ Do you realize that doctors have different ways of assessing and treating brain injury? Some are more conservative than others at deciding when a patient has advanced a level on the Rancho Scale. [See page 154.]

___ Are you prepared for your survivor's potentially disturbing transition from her coma [see page 59] to full consciousness? You may want to limit visits during this time.

___ Are you aware that when your survivor awakes she may not recognize and trust you?

___ Your survivor may confabulate or perseverate. See page 162 for descriptions of these two common behaviors when someone emerges from a coma.

___ Do you know that recovering from a brain injury is not a straight process? Your survivor likely will experience setbacks in her recovery and rehabilitation.

___ Are you aware that three parties—your doctor, the health insurance company, and the rehabilitation facility—determine the next step in your survivor's recovery: inpatient rehabilitation, a skilled nursing facility, or home? [See page 155.]

___ Do you know that there are six types of impairments your survivor may suffer due to her brain injury?

- Physical [See page 159.]
- Cognitive [See page 160.]
- Communication [See page 163.]
- Emotional [See page 164.]
- Behavioral [See page 164.]
- Social [See page 166.]

___ Do you understand that there is a powerful cause and effect relationship among these impairments? Do you know the difference between primary and secondary impairments? If not, see page 158.

___ Do you know that spasticity [see page 167] and seizures [see page 169] are common physical symptoms of a brain injury?

___ Your survivor may have difficulty communicating with you and others. Communication impairments have many different causes. Some are listed on page 163.

___ Are you prepared for some emotional distress and possible behavioral problems as your survivor adjusts to her new condition? The more common emotional and behavioral complaints are shown on pages 164 and 165.

___ Do you know that loneliness is a very common complaint of people living with a brain injury? Social impairments are discussed on page 166.

___ Are you aware that a brain injury places enormous stress on the family? For ideas on handling this stress see page 173.

___   Have you thought about how your children will cope
       with this family crisis? Some suggestions for making
       this time easier for them are presented on page 174.

___   What should you tell your children about your family
       member's brain injury? This also is discussed on page
       175.

___   Should your children come to the hospital to visit your
       survivor? This question is addressed on page 176.

___   Your older children may want to participate in the care
       of your loved one. Some ways for them to help are
       listed on page 177.

___   Do you understand that the presence of a family
       member or a close friend during rehabilitation will
       motivate your survivor to work harder? Will you be
       able to perform this important job? You may want to
       ask family members and friends to clear their schedules
       to attend some rehab sessions with your survivor. [See
       page 197.]

13

In Limbo
Stranded between Intensive Care and Rehabilitation

Jessica's condition was improving. She no longer required the specialized care of the Intermediate Care Unit, but Dr. Thomas still believed she wasn't ready for rehabilitation. So Jessica was parked in limbo, a regular ward in the hospital, where the nurses had too many patients and too little expertise in brain injury. I was worried.

My fears were soon realized. On her first morning in limbo, Jessica finally succeeded in pulling out an IV that had been annoying her for a week. If this had occurred the day before in the IMC, the IV would have been replaced immediately. In limbo, it took nearly two hours. Later that day, when I returned to her room after a quick lunch, I found Jessica lying in soiled sheets.

I was angry and I soon realized that Jessica also was angry, in a manner I had not yet seen. At the time, I thought her anger was just a new symptom of her confusion. In fact, it was the birth of a phenomenon that has lasted more than eleven years.

Jessica unconsciously mimics my mood. Three weeks passed before I recognized this. If I had connected the dots sooner, I could have spared Jessica some unnecessary grief by stepping outside when my emotions got the better of me.

At this time, only Jessica's sister, Barbara, and I had gained a small portion of Jessica's trust. Barbara accomplished this through sheer stubbornness. She spent hours at the hospital, holding Jessica's hand, repeatedly identifying herself.

Jessica was still agitated much of the day. When in a frenzy, she was difficult to control. We discovered that she enjoyed having her face washed and we kept a cool wet cloth nearby.

That night, before going to bed, I worried about how Jessica would manage her first night in limbo when she was alone and agitated. She panicked easily and didn't yet have the awareness to press the call button for help. Her nurses assured me that with her medications Jessica would sleep through the night. They also promised to check on her regularly.

The image of Jessica alone, frantic, and restrained got me to the hospital especially early the next morning. When I reached Jessica's room, she was desperately trying to scratch an itchy nose. Her arms and legs were tied to the bed railings. She had wiggled into a corner and was so entangled in the restraints she couldn't move. I freed her arms and legs and tried to hold her, but she was inconsolable. After about fifteen minutes of a slowly subsiding fury, she fell asleep, exhausted from her frustrated efforts to relieve an itch, and her first steps toward learning to live with a brain injury.

This was, perhaps, the lowest point in my perpetually fluctuating emotions: grief versus joy, despair versus hope, resignation versus determination. I couldn't spend day and night with Jessica. I had to trust the nurses who promised to check on her more often. I also couldn't help but question my optimism; perhaps Anita was right. Was the future inevitably grim? But then the day brightened.

That afternoon, Barbara was sitting with Jessica when Karen, a physical therapist, moved Jessica's arms and legs through range-of-motion exercises to guard against spasticity. When Karen worked on Jessica's left side—the one that bore the brunt of the collision—Jessica grimaced with pain. She kept looking at Barbara as if to say, "Make her stop; this really hurts."

When Karen finished her work, she asked Jessica to say goodbye. At first, Jessica just stared uncomprehendingly at Karen, who repeated her request four times. Then, to Barbara and Karen's surprise, Jessica moved her lips as if to say "Bye." They were as delighted as a mother hearing her child's first words.

Rehabilitation is akin to an accelerated infancy and childhood. The survivor may have to rediscover a lifetime of acquired skills. Fortunately, much of this information still is lodged in her damaged brain, but the pathways to it have been disrupted. Much of rehab is developing new connections in the brain through the guided rehearsal of the skills being re-taught. A patient relearns how to dress herself with the guidance of a trained therapist who leads her through each step until the skill again has been mastered.

Occasionally, Jessica was able to relax and trust the people around her. This was another sign that her recovery was moving forward. Her sweet and caring side somehow asserted itself through the fear, pain, and anxiety afflicting her much of the time. In these moments, she held her arms out wide for a hug and gently patted the back of whoever accepted the invitation.

Jessica also passed through a brief phase of kissing the hands of just about everyone who paraded through her room: family, friends, nurses, doctors, therapists, even the men and women who brought her meals. Certain people were thrown by this childlike gesture. Dr. Thomas withdrew his hand in embarrassment. Dr. Stevens took Jessica's hand and ceremoniously held it to his lips.

The decision—where would Jessica go next: an inpatient rehabilitation facility or a nursing home—had to be made in the next few days and we were anxious to hear from Dr. Thomas. The call finally came when I was home soaking my sore muscles in a hot bath. At last, Dr. Thomas recognized Jessica's progress and declared her ready for rehab. We should now engage Jessica more often, he instructed. "Talk to her, read to her, or play music every three hours for up to fifteen minutes," he said. "But stop if she becomes agitated or falls asleep."

When I pressed him for a long-term prognosis—this was our final conversation—Dr. Thomas hemmed and hawed. When I persisted, he said, "I think she'll eventually be able to go home, but she'll need a lot of help. You may need to hire someone to help care for her. But it's really too soon to tell." By then I knew Dr. Thomas well enough to recognize that he was giving me his worst-case scenario. So, on the twenty-third day of her recovery, Jessica officially reached *Level 4: Confused-Agitated* on the Rancho Scale.

> **Level 4: Confused-Agitated.** The patient is alert and restless. She's confused because she doesn't understand what's happened to her. Her attention span is short. Her behavior is without purpose and can be bizarre. She may cry out or try to remove her feeding tube. She can be hostile and uncooperative.

Jessica's story illustrates how recoveries routinely deviate from the progression of the Rancho levels. In certain areas, Jessica's actions matched *Level 4*. She was agitated. When awake, she was in constant motion. In brief moments, she surpassed *Level 4*. She was aware of the good intentions of the people around her as shown by her hugs and kisses. However, in a few ways, she had not yet reached *Level 4*. We still had bizarre, hostile, and uncooperative behavior to look forward to.

When it had become clear that Jessica would survive her brain injury, I began to consider which items on the unpalatable menu of potential impairments she might suffer as a consequence of her car crash. We had a solid, loving twenty-year relationship, but I couldn't help but worry that we, as a couple, might not survive Jessica's brain injury. I gathered from my reading that marriages frequently dissolve under the challenges of living with a brain injury. As Jessica's doctors gave me few clues as to what this "new Jessica" might be like, I couldn't help but dread a lifetime of caring for a woman I no longer loved.

What challenges would we face, I wondered?

The impairments caused by a brain injury can be grouped any number of ways. As I discussed earlier, I prefer to use six categories: physical, cognitive, communication, emotional, behavioral, and social.

I was confident that Jessica and I could cope with any physical problems. We had learned to live with my chronic pain, which disables me in many ways.

As to cognitive complaints, after three weeks of reading about brain injury, I had accepted the near certainty that Jessica would be unable to return to her job. A blow to the brain wreaks havoc on those skills—memory, planning, trouble-shooting, and problem-solving—essential to Jessica's profession. I also doubted whether Jessica would be able to work at any job. This was okay. Financially, we had been prudent savers, and our disability benefits would cover most of our expenses.

I also wasn't overly concerned about communication difficulties. Don't they say that two people who have been together for a long time finish each other's thoughts and sentences? We hadn't yet reached that degree of telepathy, but we knew each other very well.

I was less comfortable with the possible emotional, behavioral, and social complaints Jessica might suffer. It certainly was possible that her personality would change dramatically. She could be troubled by any of a wide range of emotional problems, such as depression, irritability, anxiety, and uncontrollable anger. She could develop any number of deviant behaviors, such as egocentricity, paranoia, physical violence toward others, and sexual disinhibition.

Any combination of these complaints could ruin Jessica's social life, scaring away old friends, and sabotaging efforts to make new ones. Being Jessica's only friend and constant companion would sap my energy and make me very grumpy. As an introvert, I need time to myself, even time away from the love of my life.

I often imagined any number of new Jessicas with varying mixes of emotional, behavioral, and social problems straining our relationship and testing the strength of my vows.

Would I love this new Jessica?

Would this new Jessica love me?

The thought of a loveless marriage—till death do us part—kept me tossing and turning at night.

14

An Introduction to Rehabilitation
The Healing Brain

My goal with this chapter is to prepare you for the next step in your survivor's recovery: rehabilitation. I begin by discussing post-traumatic amnesia, a state of awareness survivors pass through on their way from a coma to full consciousness. Many survivors, when they begin rehabilitation, are going through post-traumatic amnesia. Next, I present an overview of the rehabilitation process, focusing on the critical role of the family. One of your responsibilities is to select a rehabilitation facility for your survivor. I offer some guidelines for making this important decision. I close this chapter with a few thoughts about nursing homes, as some survivors will be placed in one of these facilities as they wait to enter a rehabilitation program.

Post-Traumatic Amnesia

When your survivor emerges from her coma, she likely will have little or no short-term memory. She may be disoriented, agitated, angry, impulsive, or extremely emotional. She may be disinhibited, demonstrating a complete disregard for social conventions. She may act like a child. She may behave bizarrely or in a manner completely alien to her personality.

This is a normal part of the healing process. It is called post-traumatic amnesia (PTA). For years, PTA was defined as the period of time after an injury when the brain is unable to form continuous day-to-day memories. More recently, the definition has been broadened to include a state of disorientation to time, place, and person. In this condition, the survivor may not understand who she is, where she is, and what is happening to her. She may be unable to recall very basic information, such as her name, your name, the season of the year, or the name of the current president.

Memory is the slowest part of the conscious mind to recover from an injury. It can be weeks or months before your survivor is able to routinely store new memories.

In general, post-traumatic amnesia lasts three to four times longer than the preceding coma. Jessica's coma lasted two to three weeks; her PTA lasted more than ten weeks.

The duration of PTA is one of the better—but still not very reliable—predictors of long-term outcome (see page 101). As the weeks of post-traumatic amnesia pass, the odds of a good recovery diminish.

While in post-traumatic amnesia, the patient is somewhat responsive, but baffled by her surroundings. She doesn't remember her daily activities. She can't think ahead. She goes robotically from place to place and from task to task as directed by her therapists. If she's able to speak, she asks the same questions repeatedly because she can't remember the answers.

She may ask, "Where have you been all day?" when you have left her bedside for just a moment.

Answer her questions with simple words and short sentences. Don't ask her questions until you are certain she will be able to respond easily. She doesn't need any additional frustration.

Your survivor may temporarily or permanently lose some memories from before her injury. A young adult, for example, may forget she finished college ten months before her injury. Or, she may not recognize family members or friends. She may develop familial connections with her medical team as she tries to understand her environment. This can be distressing to unrecognized and ignored family members. It is usually temporary.

When Jessica became more lucid toward the end of her post-traumatic amnesia, she couldn't recollect from day to day that I had stopped working eighteen months prior to her accident. She continually worried that I would return to work— leaving her alone, perplexed, and scared—despite frequent reminders that I was retired.

During this period of disorientation, the patient can become extremely agitated and resist attempts to calm her. This is understandable. Just imagine what she's going through. She is unconsciously and frantically trying to sort through a lifetime of experiences and reconcile them with her current infant-like condition. Some patients become aggressive and uncontrollable and must be medicated to calm down. Others become psychotic, experiencing delirium and/or hallucinations.

Survivors in PTA also may confabulate. They are utterly confused by their situation. Seeking some explanation for their plight, they may mix imagination and memory to create a sometimes fantastic scenario. This scenario will probably make little sense to you, but will temporarily satisfy your survivor's unconscious need to find some logic behind her confusion. For example, many survivors imagine that the doctors and nurses are guards, imprisoning them for bad behavior, such as swearing or striking visitors.

The transition from coma to PTA can be joyful as well as painful for the family. The patient, previously motionless, now is moving and may be speaking. Everyone is relieved; their worst fears have vanished.

The patient's behavior, however, is childlike at best and, often, totally out of character. For the first time, visitors can see just how far their survivor has to recover. They are alarmed and cannot help but panic at the prospect of a grim future.

The first two weeks of Jessica's PTA were my most challenging days. With a grimace of pain and bewilderment on her face, she writhed about her bed, moving incessantly with no destination in mind. She had no idea who I was. She was unappreciative of my attempts to help her.

I don't remember ever feeling so helpless and alone. After sitting with Jessica for an hour or two, I ached for someone, anyone, to relieve me at her bedside. And once they arrived, I often fled, hoping that a short break would help me regain my optimism and fortitude.

Eventually, as Jessica gradually began to comprehend her new world, we found ways to calm her. At first, she viewed any physical contact as punishment. Since she was always trying to free herself from the tubes and lines tormenting her, we had to restrain her arms, which infuriated her.

But then something clicked and she remembered that holding hands and hugging were good things. Her behavior, however, was exasperatingly inconsistent. She was sweet and serene one moment, frantic and combative the next. I never knew what to expect.

Slowly, Jessica's disorientation and fear eased and she grew to trust that I was a good guy. Though, she had no idea I was her husband or even understood the concept of marriage.

When a person is experiencing PTA in the early days of her rehabilitation, she is able to learn some new things, including:

- Skills that require limited attention
- Activities that can be learned through repetition
- Motor skills
- Self-care activities
- Mobility and locomotion

In addition, some behavioral problems can be addressed with success during post-traumatic amnesia.

With patience and persistence, you can guide your survivor through the fog of PTA. Be careful, though, and do not confront or argue with her. Consistent behavior and steady assurances are important. Determining when your actions won't agitate your survivor takes some practice. Often, especially in the early stages, the best environment for the patient is little or no stimulation.

Here are some guidelines to follow when your survivor is in the throes of post-traumatic amnesia:

- Always identify yourself when you enter her room.
- Tell her that it is morning, afternoon, or evening, to help her orient to time.
- Warn her when you are going to touch her.
- When she trusts you, talk about her favorite things and pleasant, shared experiences.
- Talk about her pre-injury life, but avoid suggesting that she will need to create a new life.
- Show her photos of familiar people.
- Surround her with familiar objects.
- Tell her she has been injured and is in the hospital. Repeat this often.
- Assure her that she is safe from harm now.
- If you're not already keeping a journal, begin now. You'll probably spend more time with your survivor than anyone else. You may be the first to spot significant changes in her behavior. Alerting her doctor to these changes makes you a valuable member of her medical team.
- Don't ask her to recall her injury. She can't and this certainly will frustrate her.

- Most importantly, be patient with your survivor. Neurological healing takes time, a lot of time. Trying to accelerate the process only will upset her.
- Don't take any of your survivor's hurtful words or actions personally. This can be a challenge, especially if she is swearing at everyone who approaches her or takes a swing at you when you try to comfort her.
- Always remember, when a person has post-traumatic amnesia, she truly does not know what she's doing and she should not be held responsible for her actions.

Rehabilitation Basics

All survivors of a serious brain injury acquire a mix of lifelong impairments, but through hard work they can regain some abilities lost to their injuries. How is this possible? As described in Chapter 4:

- The brain begins to heal once the patient's condition is stabilized.
- Damaged—but not dead—brain cells or neurons repair themselves.
- The brain rewires itself, growing new pathways among the billions of still-healthy neurons.
- Through a process called plasticity, healthy portions of the brain assume some of the functions previously performed by the injured areas.

This spontaneous recovery is not sufficient, though, to enable a patient to reach her full post-injury potential. For the best possible outcome, your survivor must participate in a specialized rehabilitation program.

In rehabilitation, your loved one will be evaluated and treated by a team of specially trained medical professionals, who will design a therapy program to treat her particular needs.

Depending on the severity of her deficits and how well she recovers, there may be three stages to your family member's rehabilitation:

1. Acute inpatient rehabilitation in a specialized facility offering a full range of therapies
2. An outpatient day program in a structured group setting with a full range of therapies
3. Individual outpatient therapy to treat more troublesome impairments

Relearning and Compensating

Rehabilitation has two primary components:

- Relearning forgotten skills
- Compensating for more enduring impairments

Much of what a survivor has learned in her lifetime still is present in her brain after the trauma. Severed connections block access to this information and the patient can't recall how to perform many activities. Through directed training and persistent practice, rehab reprograms the brain, establishing new connections among these still-present pockets of information, enabling the patient to reacquire forgotten skills.

Jessica had to relearn, not just how to dress herself, but even how to move from a prone to a sitting position. With the support of her therapists, Jessica gradually relearned her *activities of daily living*, also known as *ADLs*, which include bathing, dressing, walking, eating, toileting, and grooming. Mastering your ADLs is the first goal in rehab. From there, the patient and her therapists work on increasingly complex activities, with one accomplishment building on another.

Despite the best efforts of your survivor and her rehab team, serious brain damage always results in some impairment that cannot be remedied. To lead a full life, your survivor must learn ways to work around her new deficits. In rehabilitation, she will be taught to recognize and compensate for her impairments.

Sometimes, compensation means a change in behavior. This is called applying *compensatory strategies*. For example, a person with a diminished memory—nearly everyone with a brain injury—is taught to keep a detailed, daily schedule to keep her from aimlessly or inefficiently passing her time.

Jessica, for example, is lost when she forgets to consult her daily planner. Before going to bed, she organizes the items she will use in the morning—medications, cosmetics, her day's schedule, and even the clothes she will wear—neatly in the bathroom. This allows her to start her day quickly and without that nagging feeling of having forgotten to do something important. When she remembers to set her alarm clock and if she climbs out of bed when it rings, her day is off to a good start.

At other times, compensation means using assistive devices, such as a watch alarm to remind the survivor to check her daily schedule, or to get ready to go to the movies. Three or four times a day, I remind Jessica to consult her daily planner or to stay focused on finishing one task before she starts two more.

Treating the Whole Person

As described in Chapter 12, a brain injury has the potential to transform your loved one in many areas: physical, cognitive, communication, emotional, behavioral, and social. Rehab is designed to treat all of these complaints.

Your survivor may have a variety of physical problems. Some may be related to the accident that caused her brain injury, such as bones fractured in a car crash. Others may be directly related to her brain injury, such as spasticity, impaired balance, or partial paralysis. A physical therapist will help her resolve, moderate, or adjust to these physical problems.

Brain trauma always upsets cognitive processes, such as memory, attention, and language. In rehab, your survivor will perform exercises to improve her memory, concentration, communication skills, and other cognitive functions.

A blow to the brain also can disturb the emotional and behavioral stability of your survivor. She may be atypically angry, depressed, or paranoid, for example. Or, she may act oddly at times: obsessive-compulsively, violently, or overly passive, for instance. A neuropsychologist or a rehabilitation psychologist will evaluate your patient and treat any emotional and/or behavioral complaints.

Finally, interacting with others in a socially acceptable manner is a learned behavior that can be skewed by a brain injury. In rehabilitation, your survivor gradually will be introduced to people: beginning with her medical team, then other hospital staff, fellow patients, and their families. When she is ready, the survivor is reintroduced into the community and her social skills are tested. A therapist may escort her to the library where she will be asked to locate books about her favorite hobby or to a restaurant where she will order lunch.

When Should Rehabilitation Begin?

In an ideal world, rehabilitation begins as soon as the survivor is medically stable. No patient should be kept in an acute hospital setting or a nursing home any longer than necessary. Combining the brain's natural healing process with rehabilitative therapy is crucial to the success of one's recovery.

We live, however, in the age of managed health care. Rehab dollars are doled out grudgingly by health insurers. Patients sometimes are limited to two weeks of inpatient rehab. Most receive only four to six weeks.

Researchers have learned that survivors benefit most from rehabilitation when they have reached *Level 3 or 4* on the Rancho Scale. One of the most agonizing times for me was helplessly watching Jessica suffer the bewilderment of post-traumatic amnesia in an acute ward of the hospital, waiting for her doctor to agree with us that she had reached *Level 4*.

The value of rehab cannot be overstated. Maddeningly, nearly all survivors do not receive all of the rehab they need to reach their maximum recovery potential. Because of this short-sighted stinginess, all of society pays in two ways: (1) the high cost of caring for a survivor who would be more independent if a few more dollars were spent on her rehab, and (2) the loss of the potential productivity of a fully rehabilitated patient.

Selecting a Rehabilitation Facility

Selecting a rehab facility is a crucial decision. It should not be rushed. There are hundreds of rehabilitation programs. They vary considerably in the philosophy, quality, and variety of the services they offer.

I was in no condition—physically or mentally—to carefully research, visit, and compare rehab facilities. I relied heavily on my sister Barbara to handle this. You may want to ask someone to help you with this time-consuming job.

To start your search, compile a list of rehabilitation facilities to consider. Ask for recommendations from the following folks:

- The hospital social worker or case manager
- The physicians treating your survivor
- Your family doctor

- Your health insurance company, as your choices may be limited by your policy
- Your state brain injury association
- Families with rehab experience
- The Brain Injury Association of America has an online searchable database which includes a list of rehab programs (800-444-6443 & www.biausa.org).
- If your employer offers an Employee Assistance Program (EAP) or a Life Events Benefit, it may include Adult/Elder Resource and Referral Services, which may help you identify facilities in your area or elsewhere.

I believe that one factor—proximity to your home—is paramount in the selection of a rehabilitation facility. As I wrote earlier, support from family and friends during rehab is an invaluable motivator for the survivor. If the rehab facility is close to home, this support role can be shared. If it's far from home, supporting the individual typically falls on just one person—usually Mom—or no one at all.

It also is easier to participate in decisions to be made about your survivor's care and to monitor the way she is treated at the rehab facility, if it's convenient for you to be there frequently.

The choice of a rehabilitation program, however, should not be based solely on location. Some folks who live in more rural areas have no choice but to travel a long way to a rehab facility.

To help you begin your selection process, here's a list of fourteen services every brain injury rehab program should have:

1. Evaluation and assessment of the patient's unique physical, cognitive, communication, emotional, behavioral, and social impairments
2. Physical therapy to regain mobility, strength, balance, coordination, and endurance
3. Occupational therapy to relearn self-care and daily living skills

4. Speech and language therapy to treat communication and swallowing disorders
5. Cognitive rehabilitation to treat deficits in attention, concentration, memory, problem-solving, planning, and decision-making
6. Neuropsychology or rehabilitation psychology to help the survivor accept the consequences of her injury and to treat any emotional and behavioral problems
7. A social skills group to relearn how to interact with others
8. Recreational therapy to relearn leisure skills and, maybe, develop new interests
9. Access to other medical specialists, such as neurologists, orthopedists, and pain management doctors, to provide treatment for other medical problems
10. Education for both the patient and the family in living with a brain injury
11. Family counseling to help everyone adjust to their survivor's impairments
12. Substance abuse counseling
13. Trips outside the rehab center to reacquaint the survivor with the community and to determine any special needs
14. Vocational therapy to help higher-functioning survivors return to work

All staff members should be well trained and experienced in treating people with brain injuries. If the facility uses students, interns, or less experienced therapists, they should be monitored closely by seasoned practitioners.

The staff of a rehabilitation facility should include:

- A *board certified* physiatrist or neurologist as the team leader
- A neuropsychologist or a rehabilitation psychologist
- Physical, occupational, speech, recreational, and vocational therapists

- A rehabilitation nurse who will assist the patient with her therapy homework in the evening and on weekends
- A clinical dietitian, as survivors often have little appetite when they begin rehab
- A case manager who will negotiate with your health insurer the duration of your survivor's therapy

When evaluating rehabilitation facilities, it's best to visit at least twice, the first time with an appointment, the second time unannounced.

Here are ten things to look for as you inspect the facility:

1. Cleanliness
2. Adequate space for many different types of therapy
3. Staff professionalism, attention, and compassion for their patients
4. Openness: Do you feel welcome observing activities, walking around, and asking questions?
5. Are the patients clean and well kept?
6. Do they appear content with their treatment?
7. Is the food appealing?
8. Is there a home orientation suite, which enables the patient to practice skills in a home setting?
9. Do you feel rushed or pressured?
10. Are there conveniences for families, such as a cafeteria, meditation room, clergy, and lounges?

Don't be swayed by how nice the facilities appear or how wonderful a brochure looks. Ask questions. Record the answers so you can compare facilities later. Consider using a tape player to record conversations and your impressions of the facility. Also, don't be shy about approaching families with patients at the facility. They are valuable sources of information.

Here are some questions to ask:

The Rehabilitation Program

- How long has the program existed?

- Is the program CARF-accredited? *The Commission on Accreditation of Rehabilitation Facilities (CARF) sets quality standards for rehab programs. If the program isn't accredited, be wary and ask why not. You can obtain a list of CARF-accredited providers by calling 866-888-1122 or at www.carf.org.*

- What is the staff-to-patient ratio?

- Are special accommodations made for special populations, such as children, seniors, and drug and alcohol abusers?

- How many people with brain injuries has the facility treated?

- How many people does the facility treat at one time?

- What is the average length of stay?

- Who determines the length of stay?

- How flexible is the program? *We were very disappointed with our program's lack of flexibility. Jessica was anxious to improve her soft and halting speech. But her request for more speech therapy and less recreational therapy—which she felt was a waste of time—could not be accommodated.*

- Does the program maintain records on patient outcomes?

- Does the facility provide outpatient rehabilitation? *This allows for a smooth transition from inpatient to outpatient therapy, which is helpful since you and your survivor will be coping with many other issues when she returns home.*

- How often will you be able to speak to the doctor who heads your patient's treatment team?

- Is it possible to get the names and contact information for three or four survivors and their families who completed the program? *I didn't do this and I wish I had. I might have been more aware of problems with the program and acted more quickly to correct them.*

- What are the program's weaknesses? What services do you not provide?

- What recourse is there if you question or disagree with the quality or necessity of services being provided?

The Role of the Family

- What role do family and friends play in the program?

- Is the family welcome to regularly attend therapy sessions? *If the answer is "No," you may want to look elsewhere.*

- What is the visitation policy? *Family and friends should be allowed to visit at any time.*

- Can a family member sleep in the survivor's room?

- Are there regularly scheduled meetings with the family? How frequently? *An initial meeting should be held to discuss the patient's impairments and rehab goals. Then, all parties should meet again at the halfway point to discuss the patient's progress. A third meeting should be held to discuss the patient's homecoming and need for additional therapy.*

- Is reading material available to educate the family about brain injury?

- If you live far away, how much telephone contact will there be with the patient and the medical staff?

- Also, what housing arrangements can be made for you?

The Rehabilitation Team

- What are the rehab team members' credentials?

- How long has each team member been on staff?

- How frequently do team members meet to discuss a patient's condition?

- Will you have access to all team members?

- How are student therapists used in the program? *Jessica frequently had a student speech therapist, who was not monitored closely by a more experienced staff member.*

Addressing Behavioral Problems

- How does the program treat behavioral problems?

- Are restraints, safe rooms, secure and/or locked rooms used? In what circumstances?

- Is the family consulted about the use of them?

Addressing Cognitive Impairments

- What approaches are used to treat cognitive deficits?

- Is neuropsychological testing used to determine the patient's core cognitive problems?

- If neuropsychological testing is not performed, how are cognitive problems diagnosed?

- How are the results of these tests used?

- Are patients retested at a later date to determine progress?

Daily Living

- What are the rights and responsibilities of the patient?

- Is there therapy on Saturday and Sunday? *Jessica had therapy only on Saturday mornings. These sessions, which were led by a junior therapist in a group setting, were a waste of time and precious health care dollars.*

- What will your survivor do in the evening and on weekends? *Jessica found Sundays unbearably boring, especially near the end of her stay when she was desperate to go home.*

- How frequently is the patient bathed?

- How many workers are on the night shift? What are their responsibilities? *Jessica dreaded nighttime. She had difficulty sleeping, was not allowed to go to the bathroom by herself, and often found the night staff indifferent to her needs. We later learned that this is common in many facilities.*

- Can the program accommodate any special cultural or religious needs?

- How does the program accommodate special diets and personal food preferences?

- Is outside food permitted for your patient? *Jessica had little appetite and was shedding pounds. I was able to tempt her a bit with her favorite foods.*

- Are conjugal visits allowed?

Discharge Planning

- How long will your survivor be at the facility?

- Who decides when inpatient rehab ends?

- How is this decision made?

- Where will your survivor go after inpatient rehab?

- What role does the survivor and family have in these decisions?

- Does the staff teach the family how to cope with their survivor's impairments when she returns home?

- Does the staff teach the family how to continue rehab at home?

- How is the patient prepared for going home?

- Will therapists visit your home and help you prepare for the special needs of your survivor?

- Will your survivor be allowed home visits before she completes the program? *Home visits provide a clearer picture of a patient's functional problems and should be used to identify therapy goals and exercises.*

- Are there follow-up services after discharge? How frequently? *We had five follow-up appointments with the doctor who headed Jessica's rehab team.*

Paying the Bills

- How much does the program cost?

- How much of this cost will your insurer pay?

- Are there any charges not covered by insurance?

- How much will you pay out-of-pocket?

- How much flexibility is there with your insurer? *We were able to obtain extra outpatient therapy sessions by agreeing to leave inpatient rehab a week early. This worked well because both Jessica and I were ready for her to go home.*

Nursing Homes

If your survivor is not yet ready for rehabilitation, but no longer requires the special care of an acute hospital, your health insurer will no longer pay the hospital bill. In this situation, you have three options:

1. You can pay the bill yourself, if a bed is available.
2. You can care for your patient at home, but this is a demanding job that requires medical skills.
3. You can place your loved one in a long-term care facility, such as a nursing home, until she's ready for rehabilitation.

Given that some nursing homes provide substandard care and most have little expertise in brain injury, this can be a chilling prospect.

According to one study, an estimated twenty to thirty percent of people hospitalized with a moderate or severe traumatic brain injury are discharged to nursing homes. Within one year, eighty percent of these survivors move to a private home, a community-based residence, an assisted living facility, or a rehabilitation hospital.

Federal and state government agencies monitor the country's approximately 17,000 nursing homes. They compile service quality information in such areas as accurately administering medications, preventing abuse or neglect, improperly using restraints, and failing to prevent or properly treat bedsores. While this information paints an incomplete picture of service quality, it will help you weed out the worst offenders.

The folks who administer Medicare (800-633-4227 & www.medicare.gov) have a service called *Nursing Home Compare*, which provides detailed information about the past performance of every Medicare- and Medicaid-certified nursing home. Each nursing home is rated on a one-to five-star system to help you compare facilities and identify areas for closer scrutiny. There are ratings in three areas: health inspections, staffing, and ten quality measures. You can learn more about this system at www.cms.hhs.gov.

Additional information on nursing homes is available from the following organizations:

- The American Association of Homes and Services for the Aging (202-783-2242 & www.aahsa.org)
- Your state's Office of Elder Affairs
- Your state's Office of Health Care Administration

The best way to evaluate a nursing home is to visit it regularly, sometimes with an appointment and sometimes without. It's also best to visit at varying times throughout the day and evening. During these visits, talk to everyone, including staff, residents, and visitors. If you feel ill at ease, you may want to look elsewhere.

Nursing homes are not the best environment for a person with a serious brain injury. If you have no other options, make the best of the situation by heeding these nine suggestions:

1. Provide the staff with short, easy-to-read material on the basics of brain injury, perhaps portions of this book.
2. If necessary, teach the staff how best to treat your loved one.

3. Be vigilant. Visit often. An overworked staff will be more likely to treat your survivor well if they know you are watching.
4. If your survivor is not getting the care she needs, keep detailed notes and take photographs to bolster your argument that she needs more attention.
5. Arrange for therapy, even if it's just range-of-motion exercises, from either in-house staff or outside therapists.
6. Remember, your objective is to have your loved one moved to a rehabilitation facility as soon as possible.
7. Stay in touch with the rehabilitation facility you have selected for your patient.
8. Be sure the attending physician and therapists document even the slightest progress in your survivor's condition.
9. Be sure a professional with specialized training in brain injury recovery examines your patient regularly to determine if she's ready for rehabilitation.

Finally, paying for nursing home care can become an issue if your survivor does not have long-term care insurance and does not qualify for Medicaid. Your health insurer will pay the bills only if your patient is regaining function.

Checklist for Success #5
Planning for Rehabilitation

____ Do you know that if your survivor is transferred to a regular ward in the hospital, she may receive inadequate care as her nurses will have little experience with brain injuries? [See page 181.]

____ Do you know that regaining the trust of your survivor, who probably will be very confused when she emerges from her coma, may require some time and effort? [See page 182.]

____ Are you familiar with post-traumatic amnesia? This is the state your survivor will likely pass through on her way back to full consciousness. Do you know how to interact with a patient in post-traumatic amnesia? If not, see page 191.

____ Do you understand how the brain heals from an injury and what role the survivor and her caregivers play in the recovery process? You may want to reread portions of Chapter 4. [See page 45.]

____ Do you know that the two major components of brain injury rehabilitation are relearning and compensation? You can read about this on page 193.

____ Do you know how to select a rehabilitation facility for your survivor? For some suggestions, see page 196.

____ Do you understand the role of the family in rehabilitation? If not, see pages 197 and 201.

___   Do you know how to select a nursing home for your survivor, if necessary? See page 206 for some advice.

___   Do you know what to watch for while your survivor is in a nursing home? If not, see page 207.

___   Do you know how to get a copy of your survivor's medical records from the hospital? You will need them for consultations with doctors for years after the brain injury. Also, these records are important evidence for health insurance, disability benefits, and legal claims. Getting a copy of these records may take some assertiveness.

15

Eleven Years Later
The Future Can Be Bright

Jessica and I are lucky. My fears of bringing home a "new Jessica," a person I would be unable to love, proved to be unfounded. The majority of Jessica's impairments are physical and cognitive, with only a few emotional and behavioral problems.

Eleven years after her car crash, Jessica still suffers from chronic pain from her fractures. This pain slows her down, but doesn't deprive her of an active life.

Cognitively, as expected, Jessica is not as sharp as she was before her injury. She can no longer work as the information management consultant who advised colleges and universities across the country. She can no longer be the cool, calm, and collected speaker at conferences, nor the multitasking expert in constant motion at her desk—simultaneously tapping on a keyboard, talking on the phone, and meeting with a colleague.

In her personal life, Jessica—a lifelong animal activist—can no longer dream of participating in major animal rescue missions like those that follow catastrophes such as Hurricane Katrina.

Despite these changes, Jessica stays busy and productive throughout the day. She drives and runs all of our household errands. She exercises regularly. She has volunteered at a hospital and a hospice. She is an active member of the vegetarian community in our university town, and she participates in a book discussion group, holding her own with the PhDs in the group.

Jessica pursues her animal rescue ambitions by volunteering at a nearby rescue sanctuary for monkeys, where she is on the board of directors. She also has turned our house into a foster home for cats, who constantly meow and demand my attention as I sit typing away at my computer.

In these many endeavors, Jessica has developed a wide circle of warm, caring, bright, and energetic friends, who through their joint activities challenge Jessica to continue her recovery every day.

Like nearly all survivors, Jessica has a poor short-term memory. She frequently forgets the day of the week. Often, at bedtime, she can't remember how she spent the day. To compensate for this, Jessica keeps a daily planner and uses notes liberally, though she sometimes forgets to read her notes.

Jessica is distracted easily. She will go to the kitchen for a cup of tea. Thirty minutes later, I'll find her straightening the cabinets. When she is tired or anxious, she is overwhelmed by even a short list of tasks. Fortunately, she has a terrific assistive device that keeps her focused and on schedule. His name is Garry.

Jessica also is unable to pace herself. She sprints through her daytime activities and then collapses onto the couch for four, five, or six hours of watching movies before going to bed.

Emotionally, Jessica had a few bursts of inappropriate anger and disinhibition in the first two years after her injury. Now, she is able to control them. Jessica also is prone to anxiety and depression, but she manages these well with counseling and medication.

The new Jessica is—and probably always will be—too quick to become angry with me, but not with others. Caregivers, take note here: It's likely only you will recognize and experience all of the transformations in your survivor. This can be exasperating when others are unable to empathize with the challenges you face. Only another caregiver truly will appreciate your predicament. Being able to vent to other caregivers in a support group can be invaluable to your mental health.

Jessica and I have two major areas of contention. Her plans for the day are regularly sidetracked by obsessive behavior. We have the neatest and cleanest garage in town and the dishes in our cabinets are precisely arranged. The pleasure Jessica takes in arranging and rearranging the garage and kitchen, and the frustration it causes me when she has no time for other activities, is a point of friction we have been unable to resolve.

Jessica also gets so caught up in living her own life, she frequently fails to recognize and respond to my needs, even when reminded. Sadly, this is a common complaint of caregivers. I must remind myself—all the time—that Jessica's brain damage, not a lack of love or compassion, is responsible for this painful oversight.

Finally, Jessica's social skills are still strong. She's warm and caring and forms friendships with everyone who crosses her path. Loneliness is not a problem for Jessica, and I have ample time to myself.

We feel fortunate. Given the gravity of Jessica's brain injury, our lives could be much worse. Jessica recognizes her impairments. She worked diligently in her rehabilitation to overcome many of them. For those complaints that stubbornly hang on to complicate our lives, we have learned to compensate for many. Jessica refuses to allow her impairments to rob her of a full and productive life.

And, if you are wondering: Yes, I love this new Jessica. And, yes, this new Jessica loves me.

This book, though, is not just about Jessica and me. It's about all survivors of a brain injury and the people who care for them. When I began my research for this project, I was saddened to discover that many longtime survivors are struggling mightily and not living satisfactory lives. Far too many feel isolated from the rest of the world. Their social contacts are limited to the people who attend their support group meetings. Their lives are far from meaningful, productive, and happy. They feel abandoned by the medical community that saved their lives. "Now what?" they ask. "How are we supposed to live with a brain injury?" Far too many survivors spend far too many hours sitting home alone watching television.

Many survivors fail to reach their fullest post-injury potential. They do so for many reasons, but four are paramount:

1. The survivor receives little or no formal rehabilitative therapy, usually due to limited health insurance.

2. Recovering from a brain injury is the hardest work you can imagine. Often, the survivor does not exert the effort needed to excel in her rehabilitation and recovery.

3. Living with a brain injury is difficult. Survivors need the understanding and support of those around them. Too often, family and friends do not provide this support.

4. Living with a brain injury takes courage. The brain must be exercised and challenged to reach its full potential, whether or not it has been injured. Too many survivors fail to challenge themselves after they return home and reenter the community.

Let's take a look at each of these four reasons.

First, as I discussed earlier, health insurers are stingy with rehabilitation dollars and most survivors do not receive as much rehab as they need. As a caregiver, your responsibility is to ensure that you have negotiated the best possible combination of inpatient and outpatient rehab services for your survivor. When formal rehabilitation ends, there are many materials you can use with your survivor at home to continue her therapy. Any activity that challenges the mind and/or the body is therapy. Two excellent sources of material designed specifically for brain injury rehabilitation are:

- Lash and Associates Publishing/Training Inc. (919-562-0015 & www.lapublishing.com)

- The Traumatic Brain Injury National Resource Center (804-828-9055 & www.neuro.pmr.vcu.edu)

Second, rehab is hard work, probably the most difficult job your survivor will ever encounter. Rewiring the brain, relearning skills developed over a lifetime, is not only difficult, it's a slow process. Consequently, successfully surviving a brain injury requires persistence and diligence.

For the survivors reading this book, it is critically important that you recognize that you can continue to recover lost abilities as long as you keep working hard at it. Don't give up. Keep trying. The rest of your life depends upon it.

For caregivers, it is important that you find ways to support and motivate your survivor in this hard work.

Prior to her injury, one of Jessica's hobbies was basket-weaving. After she completed her formal rehabilitation, she decided to make a basket for my sister Barbara to thank her for the weeks she spent with us immediately after Jessica's accident. What would have been an easy task prior to Jessica's injury was maddeningly difficult for the new Jessica. A few times, she threw the basket to the ground in frustration. Each time, however, she picked it up and figured out what to do next.

Third, it is essential that the people important to the survivor, understand that she has been altered in many ways. This kind of permanent transformation is disturbing, if not devastating, not only for the survivor, but also for the people important to her: spouses, parents, siblings, children, friends, and co-workers. These people must not only acknowledge her new deficits, they must learn how to work with her to accommodate them.

I have seen far too many recoveries fail because the survivor's significant others—even their own family—are unable or unwilling to acknowledge and learn to live with the unwelcome changes brought about by their loved one's injury.

Our friend, George, for instance, is alienated from his family. They made little effort to understand his condition and continually accused him of malingering. "Why do you keep blaming your difficulties on something that happened years ago?" they asked, one time too many.

George also received poor performance reviews at work because his unsympathetic boss refused to make the few accommodations George needed to be a productive employee.

George's story is heartbreaking. Far too often, the families and friends of survivors prove to be obstacles rather than supporters of a successful recovery.

Finally, recovering successfully from a brain injury requires courage. Survivors often are uncomfortable with the changes in their capabilities. They fear failing in front of family, friends, and strangers. They choose to stay home and not challenge themselves.

Soon after we moved to Gainesville, Jessica was invited by her cousin to join a professional women's club. When Jessica walked onto the stage to introduce herself to the 120 members, she broke into tears as she struggled to find the words to describe her brain injury and the person she was prior to her accident. In time, though, Jessica became a valued member of the group, participating in many of their altruistic activities.

Jessica also bravely introduced herself to the founder of Jungle Friends Primate Sanctuary. She spoke of her love of animals and her willingness to work hard. Over the years, Jessica has cut vegetables for the monkeys' meals, participated in fundraising, written thank you notes to contributors, cleaned habitats, and hand-fed ailing monkeys.

Most people don't understand the long-term consequences of a brain injury. They don't realize that survivors must contend with a wide range of disabilities. All too often, they allow these disabilities to make them uneasy.

Caregivers, it is your responsibility to ensure that the people surrounding your survivor understand the difficulties she is facing and are shown how they can work with her to accommodate them.

Survivors, it's your responsibility to take chances, to push yourself beyond your current capabilities; this is the only way you will regain some of your lost abilities. This is not easy, but it is essential to rebuilding a full and productive new life.

Caregivers also have a responsibility to themselves. Caregiving can be exhausting. Exhaustion can lead to illness. An ill caregiver is a poor caregiver. It is that simple.

Caregivers, you must take periodic vacations from caregiving, even if it is only for an hour or a day. Though, one or two weeks are preferable.

Survivors, it is your responsibility to encourage your caregiver to take these vacations, and to be understanding and supportive when they suggest them. Jessica is usually hurt when I first mention a vacation on my own, but after a night's reflection she becomes supportive.

The future can be bright for people who have acquired a brain injury. This bright future, however, is achieved only through hard work, understanding, and compassion by both the survivor and those surrounding her.

Notes

Glossary

(Italicized words are defined in this glossary.)

Academy of Certified Brain Injury Specialists (ACBIS): a voluntary national certification program for professionals working in the field of brain injury.

Acceleration-Deceleration Brain Injury: a type of *closed head brain injury* that occurs when the body experiences a sudden acceleration or deceleration. This can have two devastating results: (1) the brain can slam against the bony ridges of the interior of the skull, and (2) *neurons* can be twisted and stretched severely, resulting in a *diffuse axonal brain injury*. See page 43.

Acquired Brain Injury: this term has two definitions: (1) any damage to the brain acquired after birth; or (2) damage to the brain caused by an internal event, such as a *stroke* or an *aneurysm*, not by an external trauma. See page 44.

Activities of Daily Living or ADLs: the basic activities people perform every day, including bathing, grooming, dressing, walking, eating, and toileting. Mastering the ADLs is the first goal in rehabilitation.

Acute Care: short-term care for an illness or injury generally provided in a hospital; distinguished from the critical care of an intensive care unit, the long-term care of a skilled nursing facility, and the therapeutic care of a rehabilitation program.

Aneurysm: a bulging, weak area in the wall of an artery supplying blood to the brain. When an aneurysm ruptures, blood pours into the skull potentially causing an *acquired brain injury*.

Anoxic Brain Injury: a form of *acquired brain injury* in which the supply of blood and oxygen to the brain is disrupted <u>totally</u> for more than a few minutes, causing severe damage.

Anterograde Memory: the ability to recall events that occur after an injury. Survivors often have lapses of anterograde memory for days or weeks after their brain injury. See page 161.

Aura: the subtle symptoms of *post-traumatic epilepsy* which may precede a moderate or severe seizure. Many survivors suffer seizures. See page 170.

Automatic Neurological Responses: those activities, such as breathing, digestion, heart beat, and arousal, that the body performs involuntarily or automatically in response to internal needs or changes in the external environment; distinguished from the purposeful acts that signal the end of a *coma*.

Axon: one of the three parts of a *neuron*, the basic building blocks of the brain. Axons transmit signals to and from adjacent neurons. Neurons and the connections among them are damaged and disrupted in a brain injury. See page 38.

Board Certified: the American Board of Medical Specialties certifies doctors via a rigorous process of testing and peer evaluation. When selecting a rehabilitation facility, it's wise to ask if the physician in charge is board certified.

Brainstem: a mass of thick nerve fibers located at the base of the brain. The brainstem connects the brain to the spinal cord and passes messages between the brain and the body. The brainstem also plays a vital role in attention, arousal, and consciousness. Damage to the brainstem can result in a *coma*. See page 41.

CARF Accredited: the Commission on Accreditation of Rehabilitation Facilities sets standards and accredits more than 12,600 rehabilitation programs. If the rehabilitation program you are considering for your survivor is not accredited by CARF, it's best to ask why not.

Case Manager: a medical professional who manages health care services and advocates for their clients. See page 98.

Catastrophic Brain Injury: this is not a clearly defined medical term. I use it to describe injuries that leave the survivor in a vegetative state or so impaired they are unable to set goals for themselves to achieve a better recovery or to improve the quality of their lives. See page 20.

Central Nervous System (CNS): composed of the brain and the spinal cord, the CNS coordinates the activities of the body via messages passing from the brain through the *brainstem* and down the spinal cord.

Cerebral Contusion: a bruise on the brain.

Cerebrospinal Fluid: the liquid that cushions and bathes the brain within the skull. See page 38.

Cervical Collar: a stiff collar typically placed on accident victims by medical personnel to stabilize the neck when there is the possibility of spinal cord damage.

Closed Head Brain Injury: a form of *traumatic brain injury* in which the skull is left intact and the damage to the brain is not visible. See page 40.

Cognition: The mental processes of perceiving, thinking, reasoning understanding, judging, learning, making decisions, and planning. It is rare when cognition is not impaired by a *serious brain injury*. See page 160.

Cognitive Rehabilitation: a set of structured therapeutic activities designed to redevelop an individual's ability to perceive, think, reason, understand,, judge, learn, make decisions, and plan.

Coma: a state of unconsciousness from which the patient cannot be awakened or aroused, even by powerful stimulation. A coma is clinically defined as an inability to follow a one-step command consistently. See page 59.

Coma Arousal Therapy: a formal, but controversial therapy in which multiple stimuli are presented to the patient in a systematic manner to rouse her from a *coma*. See page 63.

Concussion: a form of *mild brain injury* usually caused by a blow to the head. A concussion may involve unconsciousness and requires rest and time to heal properly. Multiple concussions can result in considerable cumulative brain damage. See page 19.

Confabulation: the confusion of imagination and memory in response to a survivor's bewilderment and fear as she emerges from a *coma*. See page 162.

Contractures: a shortening of a muscle or a tendon in response to extreme physical stress, such as constant *spasticity*.

Custodial Care: non-medical care assisting individuals with their *activities of daily living*. It typically is not covered by health insurance.

Diffuse Axonal Brain Injury: a form of *traumatic brain injury* in which multiple areas of the brain and a vast number of *neurons* are damaged. See page 43.

Disinhibition: a lack of restraint and a disregard for social conventions, safety, and security. Disinhibition is a common brain injury symptom.

Edema: the medical term for swelling or an abnormal accumulation of fluid. The swelling of injured brain tissue contributes to *intracranial pressure* following an injury. See page 41.

Email or Internet Support Group; a support group conducted through the exchange of emails among the members for the purpose of mutual support and education. See page 232.

Executive Functioning: a loosely defined package of higher-level *cognitive* abilities responsible for planning, performing, and evaluating multi-step activities. Executive functioning often is impaired by a brain injury. See page 162.

Foley Catheter: a thin tube inserted into the bladder to drain urine.

Gastric or G Tube: a tube inserted through the abdomen and directly into the stomach for the supply of liquid nutrition.

Glasgow Coma Scale: a universal, quick, and easy-to-calculate measure of the gravity of a brain injury. See page 57.

Hematoma: the medical term for a collection of blood outside the blood vessels. A hematoma generally is the result of a *hemorrhage* or internal bleeding. A hematoma within the *meninges* can press into the brain and damage *neurons*. See page 40.

Hemorrhage: the medical term for bleeding. The hemorrhaging of injured brain tissue can create *hematomas,* which can contribute to dangerous levels of *intracranial pressure* and *secondary damage* to the brain. See page 41.

Herniation: an abnormal protrusion. With a brain injury, the brainstem can be jammed down into the vertebrae with potentially catastrophic results. See page 42.

Hypoxic Brain Injury: a form of *acquired brain injury* in which the supply of blood and oxygen to the brain is disrupted partially for more than a few minutes.

Intracranial Pressure or ICP: the level of pressure within the skull. The swelling and bleeding of injured brain tissue creates intracranial pressure within the finite confines of the skull. This pressure, if not controlled, can cause *secondary damage*, resulting in a considerably poorer recovery or even death. See page 40.

Intracranial Pressure or ICP Monitor: a device drilled into the skull to measure the level of *intracranial pressure*. See page 43.

Involuntary Neurological Responses: those activities, such as breathing, digestion, heart beat, and arousal, that the body performs involuntarily or automatically in response to internal needs or changes in the external environment; distinguished from the purposeful acts that signal the end of a *coma*.

Leave Sharing: a program in which colleagues donate vacation time to those who have a medical emergency themselves or within their family. See page 125.

Medicaid: a joint federal and state health insurance program that assists low-income people who do not have health insurance or who have exhausted their benefits. See page 120.

Medicare: the nation's largest health insurance program for individuals sixty-five years of age or older who have contributed to Social Security for a certain number of years. Medicare benefits also are paid to people who have received *Social Security Disability Income* for two years. See page 121.

Meninges: a system of membranes that envelops and protects the brain. A collection of blood or a *hematoma* within the meninges can exert pressure on the brain causing further harm. See page 38.

Mild Brain Injury: an injury with a *Glasgow Coma Scale* score of 13 or higher. See pages 19 and 58.

Minimally Conscious State: a level of consciousness in which there is minimal but definite behavioral evidence of an emerging self-consciousness and/or awareness of the environment. See page 63.

Moderate Brain Injury: an injury with a *Glasgow Coma Scale* score of 9 through 12. See pages 19 and 58.

Motor Skills: gross motor skills involve the productive use of the large muscles of the body, enabling functions such as walking, kicking, sitting upright, lifting, and throwing. Fine motor skills involve the small muscles and allow activities such as the manipulation of small objects, writing, and sewing. Motor skills often are impaired by a brain injury.

Nasogastric or NG Tube: a tube threaded through the nose or mouth, via the swallowing passage or the esophagus, and into the stomach for the supply of liquid nutrition.

Neurologist: a doctor who specializes in the diagnosis and treatment of nervous system disorders, including diseases of the brain, the spinal cord, nerves, and muscles.

Neurons: the core components of the brain, which retain, process, and transmit information via electrochemical signaling. See page 38.

Neuropsychological Testing: a formal method of determining the brain's capacity to support short and long-term memory, attention, concentration, abstract reasoning, *executive functioning, motor skills* and other *cognitive* and psychological activities. Neuropsychological testing is used to help doctors and therapists identify a survivor's core deficits and to design an effective rehabilitation plan.

Neuropsychologist: a medical professional who studies dysfunctions of the brain and how they impact behavior.

Neurosurgeon: a doctor who performs surgery for injuries and diseases affecting the brain, the *brainstem*, and the spinal cord.

Neurotransmitters: chemicals that relay, amplify, and modulate signals among *neurons*. See page 38.

Occupational Therapist: a medical professional who helps disabled clients redevelop their ability to perform their *activities of daily living*.

Open Head Brain Injury: a form of *traumatic brain injury* in which an external force tears open the scalp, cracks the skull, rips apart the *meninges*, and pierces the brain. See page 41.

Orthopedist: a doctor who specializes in the diagnosis and treatment of disorders of the bones and joints.

Peer Mentors: experienced survivors and caregivers who provide informational and emotional support to those who are new to brain injury. Your state brain injury association (see page 234) may be able to assign you a peer mentor.

Perseveration: the uncontrollable repetition of a particular response, such as a word, phrase, or gesture, despite the cessation of the stimulus that triggered the response. See page 162.

Physiatrist: a doctor of physical medicine and rehabilitation, who typically serves as the leader of a rehabilitation team.

Physical Therapist: a medical professional who evaluates and treats clients who have difficulty moving parts of their body.

Plasticity: the ability to be shaped or molded; the ability of the healthy portions of the brain to assume some of the functions previously performed by the damaged areas. See page 46.

Pneumonia: an inflammatory illness of the lungs characterized by coughing, chest pain, fever, and difficulty breathing. Survivors who have been on a ventilator for weeks or more are vulnerable to pneumonia.

Post-Traumatic Amnesia (PTA): the period of time after an injury when the brain is unable to form continuous day-to-day memories and the survivor is disoriented to time, place, and person. All survivors pass through PTA on their way back to full consciousness, some for a minute or two, others for weeks or months. See page 187.

Post-Traumatic Epilepsy: a condition of seizures occurring after a trauma, such as a brain injury. About ten percent of survivors develop post-traumatic epilepsy and experience continuing seizures of varying severity. See page 169.

Primary Impairment: an impairment that is directly related to brain damage. See page 158.

Rancho Los Amigos Scale of Cognitive Functioning: a tool widely used to classify and track a brain injury patient's degree of functioning. See page 64.

Rehabilitation Psychologist: a medical professional who helps clients—patients, family members, and caregivers—who are struggling with the effects of a disability and are seeking to rebuild their lives.

Retrograde Memory: the ability to recall events that occurred prior to an injury. Survivors sometimes have temporary or permanents lapses in retrograde memory. See page 161.

Secondary Brain Damage: the damage to the brain that occurs after the initial injury, usually caused by high *intracranial pressure*. See page 42.

Secondary Impairment: an impairment that develops as a consequence of one or more *primary impairments*. See page 158.

Serious Brain Injury: not a formal medical term. I use it to identify those injuries that fall between the mildest of *mild brain injuries* and *catastrophic brain injuries*. See page 20.

Severe Brain Injury: an injury with a *Glasgow Coma Scale* score of 8 or lower. See pages 19 and 58.

Social Security Disability Income: a monthly financial benefit available to people who are disabled for at least twelve months and have paid into Social Security for a certain number of years. See page 125.

Spasticity: a condition of abnormally increased muscle tone or the shortening and/or tightening of soft tissue muscles, tendons, and ligaments. Spasticity is a common symptom of serious brain injuries. See page 167.

Speech-Language Pathologist: see speech therapist.

Speech Therapist: a medical professional who assesses, diagnoses, treats, and helps to prevent disorders related to speech, language, communication, voice, swallowing, and fluency.

Stroke: a form of *acquired brain injury* in which there is an interruption in the supply of blood to the brain.

Supplemental Security Income: a federal and state government needs-based income program for the aged, blind, and disabled who have limited income and few financial assets. See page 131.

Tracheotomy or Tracheostomy: a minor surgical procedure in which an opening is cut in the neck, allowing the tube from a *ventilator* to be placed directly into the windpipe, rather than through the patient's mouth. A tracheotomy often is performed on survivors who have been in a *coma* for more than a few days or weeks.

Traumatic Brain Injury or TBI: a form of brain injury in which an external event or object, such as a car collision, a bicycle accident, a gunshot wound, a fall, or an assault, causes the injury. See page 39.

Vegetative State: a condition in which an individual performs no conscious or purposeful acts, such as a survivor in a *coma*. This term is usually not used until the patient has been unconsciousness for months. See page 63.

Ventilator: survivors often are unable to breathe on their own after their injury; a ventilator, also called a respirator, helps a survivor breathe via a tube that is threaded through the survivor's mouth to her breathing passage or trachea in a process called intubation.

Wake Up Response: the body's ability to move from unconsciousness to consciousness; an *automatic neurological response* that often is disrupted by a brain injury.

List of Essential Resources

There are hundreds of brain injury organizations, Web sites, and books. I have reviewed many of them and cite below what I believe are the best resources for your next step in learning about brain injury.

The Brain Injury Association of America

The BIAA is the leading national organization serving and representing individuals, families, and professionals who are touched by brain injury. Together with its network of state affiliates (see page 234) and hundreds of local chapters and support groups across the country, the BIAA provides information and support to survivors and their families. Of special interest is the National Directory of Brain Injury Services, which lists a wide range of brain injury professionals and programs.

800-444-6443   www.biausa.org

BrainLine.org

BrainLine is a national multimedia project offering information and resources about preventing, treating, and living with a brain injury. It includes a series of Webcasts, electronic newsletters, and an extensive outreach campaign in partnership with national organizations concerned about brain injury.

703-998-2020   www.brainline.org

Traumatic Brain Injury Outreach Center

The Traumatic Brain Injury Outreach Center is a telephone outreach program operated by the U.S. Department of Defense. The 24/7 phone line is staffed by behavioral health consultants and nurses, who provide information and referrals for health care resources to military service members, veterans, their families, and civilians.

866-966-1020

Defense and Veterans Brain Injury Center

The DVBIC serves active duty military, their dependents, and veterans with brain injury through state-of-the-art medical care, innovative clinical research initiatives, and educational programs. Information is available in Spanish.

800-870-9244   www.dvbic.org

The National Resource Center for Traumatic Brain Injury

The mission of the NRCTBI is to provide practical information for professionals, persons with brain injury, and family members. With more than two decades of experience investigating the special needs and problems of people with brain injury and their families, NRCTBI offers a wide variety of helpful materials for survivors and caregivers through their Web site and catalog.

804-828-9055   www.neuro.pmr.vcu.edu/catalog

Lash & Associates Publishing/Training Inc.

Lash & Associates produces and sells practical and user-friendly books, manuals, tip cards, and tool kits that describe the symptoms, treatment, and recovery of individuals with brain injury. The company also develops and presents on-site, specific, in-depth programs on traumatic brain injury and concussion in children and adults.

919-562-0015   www.lapublishing.com

Brain Injury Family Resources Blog

The mission of BIFR is to help family members of brain injury survivors by providing encouragement, advice, information, and resources in a supportive community.

www.braininjuryfamily.net

Medline Plus

Medline Plus is a service of the U.S. National Library of Medicine and the National Institutes of Health. The Medline Plus Web site provides authoritative information about brain injury and caregiving produced and compiled by U.S. government agencies and health-related organizations. The site also provides easy access to medical journal articles and has extensive information about drugs, an illustrated medical encyclopedia, interactive patient tutorials, and the latest health news.

www.nlm.nih.gov/medlineplus/traumaticbraininjury.html
www.nlm.nih.gov/medlineplus/caregivers.html

Brain Injury News and Information Blog

This blog, which is authored by Michael V. Kaplen Esq., an attorney specializing in representing people with a brain injury, provides the latest news and information on brain injury, concussion, coma, traumatic epilepsy, and other brain trauma. You can subscribe to this blog at his Web site.

www.BrainInjury.blogs.com

CaringBridge

CaringBridge offers free Web sites that support and connect family members and friends during critical illnesses, treatment, and recovery. This is an easy way to keep everyone up to date on your survivor's progress.

www.CaringBridge.org

Support Groups

One of the best ways to learn about brain injury is to join a support group. These groups typically have members who have lived with brain injury for years and understand very well what you're going through.

Not only will you gain valuable practical information, you also will receive invaluable emotional support and understanding.

If you prefer to attend a local support group, check with your state brain injury association (see page 234) for a list of the support groups in your area.

If you are more comfortable seeking support online, here are some Web-based support groups:

- www.tbinet.org
- www.tbihome.org
- www.48friend.org
- www.dailystrength.org/c/Brain-Injury/support-group
- http://brain.hastypastry.net/forums/
- http://groups.yahoo.com/search?query=brain+injury
- www.braininjurychat.org
- www.avbi.org

Books

(For short reviews of these books and others
as they are published, please visit our Web site
www.BrainInjurySuccess.org.)

Family Guides

Mindstorms: The Complete Guide for Families Living with Traumatic Brain Injury by John W. Cassidy, M.D. with Karla Dougherty, Da Capo Press, 2009

Head Injury: The Facts by Audrey Daisley, Rachel Tams, and Udo Kischka, Oxford University Press, 2009

Missing Pieces: Mending the Head Injury Family by Marilyn Colter, ColterWorks Publications, 2004. (www.braininjuryfamily.net)

Stories Written by Survivors

Cracked: Recovering after Traumatic Brain Injury by Lynsey Calderwood, Jessica Kingsley Publishers, 2003

Every Good Boy Does Fine: A Novel by Tim Laskowski, Southern Methodist University Press, 2003

I'll Carry the Fork: Recovering a Life after Brain Injury by Kara Swanson, Rising Star Press, 1999

TBI Hell: A Traumatic Brain Injury Really Sucks by Geo Gosling, Outskirts Press, 2006

Stories Written by Caregivers

Being with Rachel: A Story of Memory and Survival by Karen Brennan, W.W. Norton, 2002

Crooked Smile: One Family's Journey toward Healing by Lainie Cohen, ECW Press, 2003

A Three Dog Life: A Memoir by Abigail Thomas, Harcourt, 2006

Where Is the Mango Princess: A Journey Back from Brain Injury by Cathy Crimmins, Vintage Books, 2000

Technical Works Written by Medical Professionals

Brain Injury Medicine: Principles and Practice edited by Nathan D. Zasler, M.D.; Douglas I. Katz, M.D.; and Ross D. Zafonte, D.O., Demos, 2007

The Brain that Changes Itself: Stories of Personal Triumph from the Frontiers of Brain Science by Norman Doidge, M.D., Viking 2007

Rehabilitation for Traumatic Brain Injury edited by Walter M. High, Jr., Angelle M. Sander, Margaret A. Struchen, and Karen A. Hart, Oxford University Press, 2005

State Brain Injury Associations

Alabama	205-823-3818		Montana	800-241-6442
Alaska	888-574-2824		Nebraska	800-444-6443
Arizona	602-508-8024		Nevada	800-444-6443
Arkansas	501-374-3585		New Hampshire	800-773-8400
California	661-872-4903		New Jersey	800-669-4323
Colorado	303-355-9969		New Mexico	888-292-7415
Connecticut	860-721-8111		New York	800-228- 8201
Delaware	800-411-0505		North Carolina	800-377-1464
Florida	800-992-3442		North Dakota	800-444-6443
Georgia	404-712-5504		Ohio	866-644-6242
Hawaii	808-791-6942		Oklahoma	405-513-2575
Idaho	888-374-3447		Oregon	800-544-5243
Illinois	800-699-6443		Pennsylvania	866-635-7097
Indiana	317-356-7722		Rhode Island	401-461-6599
Iowa	800-444-6443		South Carolina	877-824-3228
Kansas	800-444-6443		South Dakota	605-395-6655
Kentucky	800-592-1117		Tennessee	877-757-2428
Louisiana	504-619-9989		Texas	800-392-0040
Maine	800-275-1233		Utah	800-281-8442
Maryland	800-221-6443		Vermont	877-856-1772
Massachusetts	800-242-0030		Virginia	800-334-8443
Michigan	800-772-4323		Washington	800-523-5438
Minnesota	800-669-6442		West Virginia	800-356-6443
Mississippi	800-641-6442		Wisconsin	800-882-9282
Missouri	800-377-6442		Wyoming	307-473-1767

Index

Academy of Certified Brain Injury Specialists, 100, 219
Acceleration-deceleration brain injury, 32, 39, 43, 44, 219
Acquired brain injury, 40, **44-45**, 219
Activities of Daily Living or ADLs, 193, 219
Acute care, 102, 116, 155, 195, 196, 206, 219
Advocating for your survivor, 13, 27, 89, 98, 106
Afghanistan war, 23, 39, 130
Aneurysm, 22, 44, 219
Anoxic brain injury, 219
Anterograde memory, 161, 219
Artery, 39, 40
Assistive devices, 67, 194, 212
Attorneys, 75, **139-144**,
Aura, 170, 220
Automatic Neurological Responses, 38, 41, 59, 63, 220
Awareness (lack of), 60, 63, 71, 75, 77, 160, 162, 164, 182, 187
Axon, 38-39, 40, 43, 220
Bedsores, 60, 207
Behavior, 27, 53, 63, 64-67
Behavioral impairments, 164-167, 185, 191, 194-195, 197-198, 203, 211
Blood pressure, 42, 43, 77, 150
Brain Injury Association of America, 13, 23, 81, 116, 141, 143, 197, **229**
Board certified, 198, 220

Brainstem injury, 34, 38, 39, **41**, 42, 48, 60, 74, 111-112, 167, 220
CARF or Commission on Accreditation of Rehabilitation Facilities, 200, 220
Caregiving
How to succeed, 79-106
Caring for yourself, 80-91
Being kind to yourself, 81
Support groups, 82
Coping with emotions, 83-91
Faith, 91-92
Asking for help, 92-95
Hiring case manager, 98-101
Hiring attorney, 139-144
Caring for your family, 171-177
During rehabilitation, 197, 201-202
Nursing homes, 206-208
Case managers, 75, **98-101**, 117, 120, 126, 190, 199, 220
Catastrophic brain injury, 20, 60, 101, 220
Central nervous system, 221
Cerebral contusion, 44, 221
Cerebrospinal fluid, 32, 38, 221
Cervical collar, 36, 110, 221
Chemicals (toxic to the brain), 40, 42, 43
Child's Benefit for Social Security Disability Income, 138
Children in the brain injury family, 92, 172-177, 216

Children with Special Health
Care Needs, 137
Children's Health Insurance
Program, 137
Closed head brain injury, 39,
40, 221
Clumsiness, 160
Cognitive impairments, 101,
129, 160-163, 168, 185, 195,
203, 211, 221
Cognitive rehabilitation, 23,
116, 121, 198, 221
Coma, 39, 41, 42, 47, 49, 55,
59-64, 71, 73, 77, 102, 109,
150, 221
Coma arousal therapy, 63, 221
Coma stimulation, **61-63**, 72
Communication impairments,
163, 185, 198
Compensation, 46, 67, 194
Compensatory strategies, 67,
194
Concentration, 20, 116, 161,
195, 198
Concussion, 19, 221
Confabulation, 162, 189, 222
Contractures, 60, 222
Counseling, 86, 89, 97, 164,
198, 212
Custodial care, 111, 139, 222
Coup contrecoup brain injury,
39, **44**,
CT scan, 44, 76, 158
Diffuse axonal brain injury, 39,
43-44, 222
Disinhibition, 159, 163, 165,
186, 212, 222
Doctors (dealing with), **54-56**
Edema (swelling), 41, 48, 155,
222

Email messages, 74, 93
Emotional impairments, 158,
164, 167, 185-187, 195, 198,
211-212
Executive functioning, 161-162,
222
Faith, **91-92**, 103
Family and friends (role of), 18,
52, 74, 90, 103, 152, 201,
214-216
Family and Medical Leave Act
(FMLA), 95-97
Family and Medical Leave Act
and Military Personnel, 97
Family guides, 81
Family impact, 171-177
Fatigue, 160, 166, 168
Focal brain injury, 39, 44, 169
Gastric or G tube, 60, 110, 222
Glasgow Coma Scale (GCS),
33, **57-59**, 102, 222
Glossary, 29
Golden hour, 33, 36
Guardianship, 56, 140
Health insurance, 24, 28, 75, 76,
85, 96, 110-111, **115-122**, 139,
197, 215
Heart attack, 22, 44
Hematoma, 40, 223
Hemorrhage (bleeding), 41, 48,
223
Herniation, 42, 43, 223
Hypoxic brain injury, 223
Impairments (primary), 158
Impairments (secondary), 158
Impairments caused by a brain
injury, 20, 39, 45, 48, 73,
157-171, 185, 217
Improvised explosive device
(IED), 39

Infection, 22, 41, 44, 60, 155
Internet support groups, 70, 222
Intracranial pressure (ICP), 33, 40, 42, 43, 47, 60, 61, 72, 77, 223
Intracranial pressure monitor, 34, 35, 36, 43, 73, 77, 223
Involuntary Neurological Responses, 59, 61, 76, 150, 223
Iraq war, 23, 39, 130
Language, 151, 158, 161, 162, 195, 198
Leave sharing, 125, 223
Level 1: No Response, 21, 52, 64, 65
Level 2: Generalized Response, 65, 72, 76
Level 3: Localized Response, 65, 154, 155, 196
Level 4: Confused-Agitated, 65, 155, 184, 196
Litany of Uncertainty, 49, 102, 111
Long-term disability, 124-125
Medicaid, 118, **120-121**, 132, 143, 146, 207, 208, 224
Medicaid for children, 137
Medicaid waiver, 121
Medicare, 118, **121-123**, 143, 207, 224
Membranes, 33, 38, 41
Memory, 19, 39, 61, 66, 67, 116, 158, 159, 161, 162, 170, 185, 187-191, 194, 195, 198, 212
Meninges, 38, 224
Mild brain injury, 19-20, 58, 128, 224

Minimally conscious state, 53, **63-64**, 224
Moderate brain injury, 19, 58, 206, 224
Motor skills, 160, 190, 224
Nasogastric or NG tube, 60, 77, 224
Neurologist, 55, 198, 224
Neurons, 38, 39, 40, 41, 44, 45, 46, 192, 225
Neuropsychological testing, 161, 203, 225
Neuropsychologist, 195, 198, 225
Neurosurgeon, 84, 225
Neurotransmitters, 38, 225
Nursing homes, 110, 122, 155, 184, 187, 195, **206-208**
Occupational therapy, 95, 116, 119, 122, 197, 198, 225
Open head brain injury, 39, **41**, 225
Orientation to person, place, and time, 66, 67, 77, 153, 162, 169, 170, 188, 189, 190, 199
Orthopedist, 55, 198, 225
Oxygen deprivation, 35, 39, 42, 43, 44, 73
Pathways, 38, 39, 41, 45, 60, 183, 192
Peer mentors, 23, 70, 164, 225
Perseveration, 162-163, 225
Physiatrist, 151, 198, 226
Physical impairments, 159-160, 195
Physical therapy, 110, 159, 183, 195, 197, 226
Plasticity, 23, 46, 192, 226
Pneumonia, 60, 74, 226

Poisoning, 44

Post-traumatic amnesia (PTA), 102, 151-152, **187-192**, 196, 226

Post-traumatic epilepsy, 169-171, 226

Privacy regulations, 56

Prognosis, 17, 49, 53, 73, 76, 102, 109, 111, 184

Purposeful acts, 21, 59, 61, 64, 67, 150

Rancho Los Amigos Scale of Cognitive Functioning, 21, 52-53, **64-67**, 72, 76, 102, 154-155, 184, 196, 226

Rehabilitation, 20, 23, 46, 52, 64, 76, 79, 80, 82, 90, 92, 95, 99, 103, 115, 116, 119, 134, 139, 151, 154, 160, 165, 168, 173, 183, **192-196**, 214

Rehabilitation (inpatient), 155, 184, 193

Rehabilitation (outpatient), 155, 193, 201

Rehabilitation and health insurance, 115-117, 215

Rehabilitation facilities, 28, 75, 196-206

Rehabilitation psychologist, 226

Relearning, 46, 183, 193, 197, 198, 215

Responding to commands, 46, 59, 61, 63-66, 76, 109, 150, 154

Restraints, 151, 182, 190, 203, 206

Retrograde memory, 161, 226

Romantic relationships, 166, 185

Safety and security, 66, 96

Second opinion, 56

Secondary brain damage, 33, 39, 40, **42-43**, 227

Seizures, 42, 160, **169-171**

Sensory impairments, 160

Serious brain injury, 20, 32, 64, 90, 123, 227

Severe brain injury, 19, 47, 58, 76, 115, 227

Severity of a brain injury, 19, 33, 57-59, 102

Short-term disability, 124

Social impairments, 166, 186, 195

Social interactions, 66, 67

Social Security Disability Income (SSDI), 75, 118, 121, **125-131**, 139

Social Security Disability Income (appealing your case), 129-131, 227

Social Security Disability Income for Children, 138

Spasticity, 60, 110, 160, **167-169**, 183, 195, 227

Speech, 20, 39, 57, 160, 163, 168, 170, 200

Speech therapy, 96, 116, 122, 198, 200, 202, 227

Spinal cord, 22, 34, 38, 110, 227

Stem cells, 23

Stroke, 22, 44, 227

Substance abuse, 22, 44, 103, 198

Success of recovery, 18, 52, 58, 90, **101-103**, 111

Successfully Surviving a Brain Injury project, 25

Supplemental Security Income (SSI), **131-132**, 227

Supplemental Security Income
  for children, 134-136
Support groups, 14, 23, 70, 82,
  103, 109, 113, 164, 213, 214,
  222, **231**
Surgery, 43, 159, 168
Tracheotomy or Tracheostomy,
  110, 151, 227-228
Traumatic brain injury, 13, 22,
  39-41, 45, 129, 228
Tumor, 22, 44
Vegetative state, 20, **63-64**, 110,
  228
Ventilator, 35, 43, 74, 110-111,
  151, 155, 228
Visitor guidelines, 69
Wake-up response, 41, 48, 74,
  228
Workers' Compensation, 118,
  132-134, 139

Brain Injury Success Books

Order Form

You can order additional copies
of this book in the following ways:

Our Web site: www.BrainInjurySuccess.org

Email: Info@BrainInjurySuccess.org

Telephone: 352-672-6672

Post: Jessica Whitmore
7025 NW 52nd Drive
Gainesville, FL 32653-7014

Book Price: $17.95

Shipping: $4.00 for the first book and $3.00 for
each additional book

Sales tax: Please add 6% for each book shipped
to a Florida address

Name: _____

Address: _____

City: _____ State: _____ Zip: _____

Email address: _____

Would you like to be added to our mailing list to be notified of
new products?   Yes   No

Would you like to participate in the *Successfully Surviving a Brain
Injury* project as a panel member?   Yes   No

Brain Injury Success Books

Order Form

You can order additional copies
of this book in the following ways:

Our Web site: www.BrainInjurySuccess.org

Email: Info@BrainInjurySuccess.org

Telephone: 352-672-6672

Post: Jessica Whitmore
7025 NW 52nd Drive
Gainesville, FL 32653-7014

Book Price: $17.95

Shipping: $4.00 for the first book and $3.00 for
each additional book

Sales tax: Please add 6% for each book shipped
to a Florida address

Name: _____

Address: _____

City: _____ State: _____ Zip: _____

Email address: _____

Would you like to be added to our mailing list to be notified of
new products?   Yes   No

Would you like to participate in the *Successfully Surviving a Brain
Injury* project as a panel member?   Yes   No

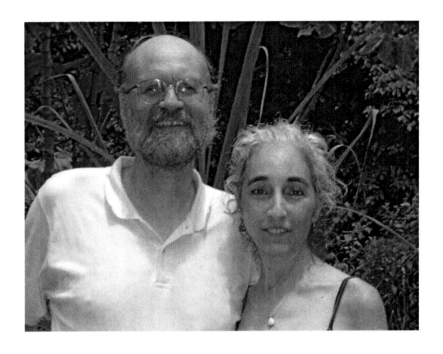

In 1997, Jessica acquired a severe brain injury in an automobile accident. Since that time, Garry and Jessica have been asking brain injury survivors, their families, and the medical professionals who treat them what it means to successfully survive a brain injury and how one achieves this success. Garry has compiled the responses collected from the hundreds of survivors, caregivers, and medical professionals, who participate in this project, into the information and advice presented in this book.

We continue to seek new participants for the *Successfully Surviving a Brain Injury* project as we examine the challenges survivors face: (1) in their rehabilitation, (2) when they return home and reenter the community, and (3) as they strive to live a full life with a brain injury. If you would like to join the panel as a survivor, a family member, or a professional, please contact us at Info@BrainInjurySuccess.org.

We look forward to hearing from you.

LaVergne, TN USA
15 September 2010
197183LV00007B/15/P

9 780984 197439